EAT PRETTY, LIVE WELL

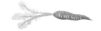

A GUIDED JOURNAL

*for nourishing beauty,
inside and out*

Jolene Hart, CHC, AADP

CHRONICLE BOOKS
SAN FRANCISCO

ISBN 978-1-4521-5192-2
Manufactured in China

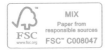

Design by Sydney Goldstein
Illustrations by Vikki Chu

The opinions expressed in this journal are solely those of Jolene Hart, a health coach
certified by the Institute for Integrative Nutrition and the American Association
of Drugless Practitioners, who is not acting in the capacity of a doctor, licensed
dietician-nutritionist, psychologist, or other licensed or registered professional. The
information presented in this book should not be construed as medical advice and is
not meant to replace treatment by licensed health professionals. Please consult your
doctor or professional health-care advisor regarding your specific health-care needs
before making changes to your diet or lifestyle.

10

Special quantity discounts are available to corporations and other organizations.
Contact our premiums department at corporatesales@chroniclebooks.com or at
1-800-759-0190.

Chronicle Books LLC
680 Second Street
San Francisco, California 94107
www.chroniclebooks.com

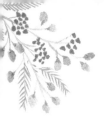

CONTENTS

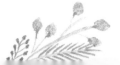

Introduction

THE POWER OF THIS JOURNAL

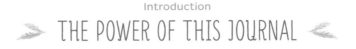

With this journal in hand, you're taking a major leap toward building a lifestyle that supports your most radiant, energetic, and beautiful self. We are living in a moment when, finally, it's recognized that beauty is more than skin deep—that it's more than a mere reflection of our skill with a makeup brush or mascara wand. Beauty comes directly from within our bodies and our selves. And we see our beauty and body at their best when we are in physical, mental, and emotional balance. This journal offers guidance, organization, opportunities for self-reflection, and support to help you find your own unique place of balanced beauty.

In my previous book *Eat Pretty,* I introduced beauty nutrition as one key to looking and feeling your best, inside and out. Beauty nutrition highlights not just the healthful benefits of foods, but their potential to enhance beauty as well—for example, cucumber contains silicon that boosts skin elasticity and moisture, and garlic has phytochemicals that block wrinkle formation. These are "beauty nutrients"—the components of your food that nourish your inner and outer beauty. In addition to linking foods to their beauty benefits, *Eat Pretty* also illustrated the deep connection between our beauty and the changing of the seasons—shifts that bring about not just environmental transitions and seasonal foods, but also new needs in our bodies and our beauty overall.

Beyond beauty nutrients, eating for beauty is also about granting ourselves the permission to enjoy food, to feel inspired by it, and to indulge in a bountiful variety. It's about no longer wasting energy and causing ourselves physical and emotional stress positioning food as our enemy when it actually has immeasurable power to bring out our most beautiful selves. After *Eat Pretty* published, I began hearing from women around the world whose lives, bodies, and relationships with food were transformed by the suggestion that food should be their greatest tool for lifelong beauty. Their success inspires me daily, and serves as a powerful reminder that small shifts in our outlook can bring about life-changing results.

Where Are You in Your Journey?

Wherever you are in your journey to build a lifestyle of beauty inside and out, there are specific sections of this journal created just for you. Here are few things to keep in mind as you welcome *Eat Pretty, Live Well* into your life.

If you read *Eat Pretty*, you learned to pack your diet with nature's most powerfully beautifying foods, transforming the way you look and feel. This journal helps take that knowledge a step further by setting goals, reinforcing new habits, and reflecting on the practices that achieve the most beautiful results for your unique body. This journal acknowledges that a diet and lifestyle supportive of optimal beauty will not be one size fits all. Use it to record your individual journey as you create your own beautiful life. It offers room to write about what's important to you, to analyze the way you care for yourself, and to focus on your goals and priorities.

If you haven't read *Eat Pretty*, this is your moment to rethink beauty—the way you look and feel every single day. You're at the very beginning of a journey that deeply connects what you see in the mirror with what you choose to put on your plate. For too long we've been stuck thinking that the only way we can get clearer skin or stronger hair is to shell out for a lineup of beauty products. While products (specifically ones that are free of harmful ingredients) are a fabulous and feel-good addition to your beauty routine, they work within the limitations of your health. The deepest, longest-lasting, and most profound changes to your beauty and body are made through your diet and lifestyle. Supercharging your meals with beautifying foods and making small adjustments to your routine affect major changes in your body. The result will be some very noticeable improvements to your beauty, head to toe, inside and out—and this journal will provide a record of your transformation.

Why a Journal?

This book is just one more element of your beautiful lifestyle. It's a practical guide packed with information, lists, and inspiration—but writing in it also creates a moment for reflection, self-love, and mindfulness. It's hard to get that same sense of self-care from reminders typed furiously on your smartphone. Apart from journaling, the only time I put pen to paper every single day is when I'm writing lists: to-do lists, grocery lists, errand lists. And while lists are unbeatable organizational tools, they don't offer the moments for reflection that you'll find in these pages.

When I finally give myself space to write my thoughts and record my habits, I'm often surprised by the results. Things get clear. I see patterns and find deeper meaning. The excess falls away, the pace of life slows, and I notice things I hadn't before. In our world of keyboards and touchscreens, it could feel a bit unnatural to pick up a pen and write your thoughts and experiences, but that's all the more reason why working through this journal is an experience to be savored.

Writing in a journal has been shown to lower stress, to improve physical and mental health, even to help you sleep better. I believe that this journal in particular amplifies those effects, by encouraging you to regularly reflect with gratitude, to find new ways to love yourself, to set transformative intentions, to discover the foods and habits that support your best self, and to devote regular time to them.

MY SUGGESTIONS FOR USING THIS JOURNAL IN YOUR LIFE:

o Jump-start a new lifestyle that could help you look and feel your best. The checklists, trackers, and reflective questions ahead are meant to inspire you to do just that.

o Record your innermost thoughts, the words that move you, and intentions for your beauty and body.

o Document your experiences as you eliminate foods that might be affecting you negatively and replace them with healthier substitutes.

o Track weeks or months of progress toward a single goal, and remind yourself to stay the course.

o Tune up or deepen your current beauty routine using the grocery lists tailored to specific beauty goals, the checklists that note the beauty foods you've tried, the pantry to-do lists, and the section to record recipes you'd like to try.

o Encourage yourself to pay closer attention to your daily habits and the way your meals make you feel by filling out the food diary.

I hope that you'll use your moments of journaling to love and care for yourself, just as you do each time you sit down to a beautifying meal.

In beauty and health,

Jolene

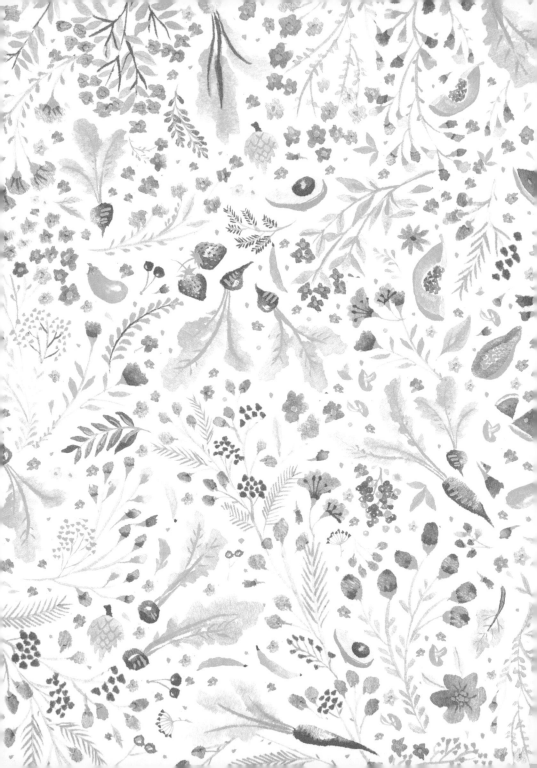

PART 1

TOOLS FOR NOURISHING BEAUTY

THE PHILOSOPHY BEHIND EAT PRETTY is that food is a more powerful beauty tool than products, treatments, and procedures combined. This approach might just bring out the skeptic in you. "I already eat well," you think, "and yet I still have an irritated complexion. My skin's just acne-prone." Or, "I'll never give up my coffee. I need it for energy, and there's no food that can deliver the boost that coffee gives me." This kind of rigid thinking prevents us from exploring new inroads into beauty, and steals opportunities to get to know our bodies better by understanding how diet and mindset truly affect us. Indeed, many of our thoughts, actions, and food choices work against our long-term beauty and health. I'm not talking about the occasional brownie—indulging now and then, and enjoying those indulgences, is essential to maintaining balance. Banning foods or adopting restrictive diets are examples of rigid approaches to beauty that only hold us back. The section ahead introduces simple shifts in outlook that, over time, can lead to significant changes in the way you look and feel. You'll also find beauty nutrition tools and guidance to help you eat pretty and live well every day.

WHAT IT MEANS TO EAT PRETTY

Food is fuel for your body, but it's never just fuel: It's social connection, emotional comfort, and physical fullness. We tend to overlook that food is also one of our greatest tools to nourish our beauty and pamper our bodies to look and feel their best—that is, if we choose our foods well. Your objective is to find the foods and habits that best support your individual beauty needs, inside and out. This journal will help you achieve that goal. The sections ahead outline the key components of what it means to eat pretty.

To Eat Pretty Is to . . . Rethink Nutrition

What makes your food choices so impactful to your beauty and body? Consider that the beauty nutrients in your food are the building blocks with which your body continually rebuilds itself, molecule by molecule, and performs the essential beauty actions of defense, repair, and detoxification. The quality of the foods you put inside your body directly influences how well your body is able to support and maintain your beauty on the outside—visible in the glow of your skin, the shine of your hair, and the energy and radiance you display head to toe.

We truly are what we eat, on a much deeper level than we appreciate. The foods that best support you in looking and feeling your best are packed with beauty nutrients, those that directly support and enhance your beauty each day by enabling actions like fighting off damage, repairing cells, and strengthening skin elasticity. By simply increasing the quantity and variety of beauty nutrients in your diet, you can prompt a change in the way your body performs, leading to physical differences—like smoother or clearer skin—that you'll see in the mirror. Maximizing the beauty nutrition in your meals has incredible potential to enhance your beauty, even more so than applying the most powerful products in your makeup bag. Remember, every time you pick up your fork, you do more than just fill a void in your stomach—you influence the way you'll look and feel tomorrow, and in the days, months, and years to come.

To Eat Pretty Is to . . . Eat for Beauty

At its core, to eat pretty is to fill your plate with the widest possible variety of foods that support beauty—those that have direct benefits to your skin, hair, nails, energy, mood, and weight—and less of the foods that make it harder for you to look or feel fabulous. But eating for beauty also means prioritizing foods that support a healthy and diverse microbiome (the community of organisms that populate your digestive system) and strong digestion, both of which are essential to break down and assimilate beauty nutrients; foods that steady your blood sugar and support hormone balance (a must-have for lifelong beauty); and foods that support detoxification, sleep, and emotional health. Focusing on the underlying processes that strengthen and reinforce wellness as a whole is a hidden key to your beauty, and a secret to building the most beautifying diet.

To Eat Pretty Is to . . . Eliminate Beauty Betrayers

Some foods appeal to your taste buds but work against your beauty by speeding up the aging process, making it harder for you to maintain a healthy weight, or sending you on a mood roller coaster. I call these foods the Beauty Betrayers. Determining which foods "betray" your beauty can be a very personal process since we all have unique associations and experiences with, as well as physical reactions to, different foods. Recognizing the effects that certain foods have on your skin, mood, and energy requires you to invest a bit more in yourself, and to look closely at your daily routine, which you will do in the fill-in trackers and self-reflection exercises in parts 2 and 3. To determine which foods benefit you and which betray you, I encourage you to work backward, looking at the processes that lead to premature aging, blemishes, common allergies or intolerances, digestive issues, hormone imbalances, and the like, as well as the foods with the greatest power to halt or reverse those processes. As you work through this journal and build your long-term lifestyle of beauty, make a conscious effort to reduce or eliminate these Beauty Betrayer foods:

Beauty Betrayers

Alcohol: This simple sugar stresses your liver (a critical organ for glowing skin), steals nutrition from your body, and disrupts your hormone balance.

Caffeine: As it temporarily boosts your energy, caffeine increases the stress hormone cortisol, which speeds up aging and wrinkling. It's an acidic compound that also prevents your body from absorbing some key beauty minerals.

Canned Foods with BPA: BPA (bisphenol-A) is an endocrine disruptor that throws off your natural hormone balance.

Dairy: A common food intolerance, dairy can fuel unwanted acne, negatively affect digestion, and add unwanted hormones to the body. If you do tolerate dairy, you may want to limit it to small amounts, and buy organic to avoid additives.

Fried Foods: Instead of healthy fats for your skin and body, these foods contain fats that are major sources of aging free radicals linked to inflammation and a host of beauty issues.

Gluten: This is another common food sensitivity that can lead to digestive issues and inflammation that wreak havoc on your skin.

Grilled and Overcooked Foods: Browning or burning food reduces its content of beauty nutrients and increases the number of age-advancing compounds inside.

Meats (Conventional): Most meat available at the supermarket is a major source of unwanted hormones and antibiotics in our diets, and is acidic and inflammatory due to its abundance of omega-6 fatty acids.

Pesticide-Sprayed Produce: Produce sprayed with pesticides increases the free radicals (associated with aging) that your body must counteract and detoxify.

Processed Foods: These are often filled with inflammatory additives, preservatives, and ingredients that offer little benefit to your beauty.

Soda: Drinking soda has links to accelerated aging, wrinkle formation, and weight gain.

Sugar: Sugar is a source of inflammation, acidity, collagen breakdown, and uncontrolled cravings—and it's addictive. Skip artificial sweeteners too, for their negative impact on blood sugar control, bloating, and cravings.

To Eat Pretty Is to . . . Cultivate Healthy Vanity

Let's rethink vanity. Too often, a focus on outward appearance and an interest in enhancing our looks is considered to be self-centered or narcissistic. Release yourself from this judgment immediately—and for good. Your goal to feel and see your beauty at its fullest potential is motivated by a quality that I call *healthy* vanity—and it's not the least bit vain. Healthy vanity is the desire to look and feel your best, and to be your best self. We all have some amount of healthy vanity within ourselves; tune into it, and let it inspire you as you build your beautiful life. Make healthy vanity your motivation to return to this journal for continual support, to add greens to your diet every day, to take the time to select fresh foods that make you feel your best, and to build a lifestyle that allows you to be as beautiful as you can be every single day.

To Eat Pretty Is to . . . Use the Seasons as Your Guide

We all experience the shifting of the seasons differently, according to our unique positions on the globe. Regardless of the degree that our winters freeze or our summers scorch, there is one constant: our environment and its seasonal changes greatly influence the needs of our beauty and bodies. By adjusting your diet and lifestyle to reflect seasonal shifts, which involves making some changes to the types of food you eat, their preparation, and to your lifestyle as a whole, you not only address cravings, you tap into your body's strengths and target your beauty needs head-on as they arise.

One example: when spring arrives, after a chilly season of eating heavier, cooked foods and often putting on some "winter weight," our body needs both cleansing and lightening. Spring delivers an abundance of fresh, alkaline greens like arugula and spinach, as well as naturally detoxifying asparagus, artichokes, and radishes, which help us cleanse and eliminate without a strict cleanse or weight loss program. I find that incorporating more of the foods that are seasonally available in your region often meets your beauty nutrition needs well enough that you experience less of the extremes that come with each season (think dry, chapped winter skin and red, sunburned summer skin).

Eating and living seasonally also helps you tap into your intuition about the needs of your beauty and body as they change throughout the year and the decades of your life. This intuitive approach to beauty and health comes from age-old, traditional wisdom that we've largely strayed from in modern times. But it's also flexible—so of course you can still eat foods out of season, since many of them are nutritious and easy to come by year-round.

There's also a major bonus to note: seasonal foods are usually cheaper, fresher, and more nutrient dense than anything grown out of season. If you're feeling a little out of touch with which foods we harvest during which times of the year, a trip to your local farmers' market lets you see, touch, smell, and taste just what the earth around you is offering your beauty right now.

To Eat Pretty Is to . . . Create a Beautifying Routine

Consistency is key when it comes to making the most positive and lasting impact on your beauty and body. The cleanse mentality— follow a rigid diet or lifestyle for a fixed amount of time, then revert to old habits—is more of a roller coaster ride than a means to greater health and balance. I strongly believe that repeating beautifying habits like sipping lemon water in the morning or carving out time for mindful breathing, simple as they may be, creates positive momentum toward major change. Seeing and feeling the benefits of your habits helps you stay committed to them, plus you're more likely to make additional tune-ups over time. In addition, you'll be able to fall back on the structure of your healthy routine when life happens— parties, splurges, vacations, cravings, and habits that could have more Betrayers than benefits. When those moments arise, enjoy them, and step right back into the beautifying life that you've built. In the pages ahead, you'll learn specific ways to support your beauty and health, which you can use to create a routine that fits your personal needs and lifestyle.

BEAUTY FOODS FROM A TO Z

This list is your go-to beauty food reference, presenting more than 150 foods, each paired with its most powerful beauty benefit. But it doesn't stop there—note that each of these foods has a multitude of benefits, so what you'll read in this section is just a taste of what these foods can help achieve in your body.

Acorn Squash:
strengthens hair and nails

Almond Milk:
boosts skin hydration

Almonds:
strengthen cell membranes

Amaranth:
supports cell repair, bone building, and strong hair and nails

Apple:
detoxifies, reduces allergies and free radical damage

Apple Cider Vinegar:
maintains pH balance, supports healthy digestion

Apricots:
support smooth skin

Artichoke:
promotes liver and gallbladder detox, and a flat belly

Arugula:
protects cells from DNA damage

Asparagus:
detoxifies, increases antiaging glutathione production

Avocado:
detoxifies, supports skin hydration

Banana:
supports healthy hair and nails, boosts mood

Basil:
protects cells from oxidative damage

Beans (black, kidney, white, etc.):
support energy, cell repair, and healthy elimination

Bee Pollen:
supports healthy digestion, energy

Beets: detoxify, increase antiaging glutathione production

Blackberries: support skin elasticity

Black Pepper: aids in nutrient absorption

Blackstrap Molasses: supports glowing skin and healthy hair and nails

Blueberries: support youthful skin and healthy connective tissue

Bok Choy: boosts production of antiaging glutathione

Brazil Nuts: help maintain skin elasticity

Broccoli: prevents stress-related inflammation

Brussels Sprouts: lower inflammation, support hormonal balance

Buckwheat: decreases wrinkle-forming compounds in the body

Burdock Root: supports healthy hair and good moods

Butternut Squash: heals and smoothes skin

Cacao: blocks wrinkle formation, reduces skin redness

Cantaloupe: protects against UV damage, maintains mitochondrial health

Cardamom: relieves indigestion, detoxifies

Carrot: heals skin, balances oil production

Cashews: support radiant hair pigmentation

Cauliflower: supports bone health and antiaging glutathione production

Cayenne: boosts immunity and metabolism

Celery: hydrates, supports healthy hair

Chamomile: promotes restful sleep and cramp relief

Chard:
strengthens hair and nails

Cherries:
prevent UV damage, support healthy connective tissue

Chia Seeds:
strengthen skin cells

Chickpeas:
support clear skin and immunity

Chives:
support healthy digestion and circulation

Cilantro:
detoxifies

Cinnamon:
moderates blood sugar spikes that lead to wrinkles and blemishes

Cloves:
aid in digestion, reduce inflammation

Coconut:
supports healthy skin, hair, and nails; protects mitochondrial health

Coconut Milk:
contains healthy fat to hydrate cells from within

Coconut Oil:
supports metabolism and fat burning

Collard Greens:
fuel skin cell repair, boost antiaging glutathione production

Cranberries:
increase blood flow to the skin, support healthy lymph flow

Cucumber:
boosts skin elasticity and moisture

Cumin:
supports digestion and healthy hair and nails

Daikon Radish:
boosts digestion and assimilation

Dandelion Greens:
maintain clear, glowing skin

Dandelion Root Tea:
supports a flat belly and liver detox

Dates:
offer low glycemic sweetness

Delicata Squash:
smoothes skin, supports healthy nervous function

Dill:
supports healthy digestion and detoxification

Eggplant:
reduces water retention, fights aging damage

Eggs (pasture-raised):
supply building blocks of beauty

Endive:
supports ovarian health

Escarole:
reduces dark circles

Fennel:
prevents inflammation, reduces UVB damage

Fennel Seeds:
boost UVB protection

Figs:
increase blood flow to the skin

Flaxseed:
detoxifies and reduces inflammation

Garlic:
blocks formation of wrinkles

Ginger:
reduces inflammation, slows cell aging

Goji Berries:
support antiaging hormone and glutathione production

Grapefruit:
protects skin from UV damage, hydrates, detoxifies

Grapes:
protect DNA health, reduce water retention

Green Beans:
promote skin strength and elasticity

Green Tea:
blocks wrinkle formation, reduces UV damage, revives dying skin cells

Hemp Seeds:
help heal eczema, excellent source of beauty protein

Honey (raw):
supports immunity and allergy reduction

Kale:
heals and clears skin, boosts cell turnover

Kimchi:
supports a healthy microbiome

Kiwi:
boosts collagen production, supports a flat belly

Kohlrabi:
supports liver detox and DNA defense

Leek:
boosts the body's antioxidant defenders

Lemon:
detoxifies, supports collagen production

Lentils:
support energy and cellular repair

Lime:
detoxifies, supports healthy collagen

Maple Syrup:
contains trace minerals that support hair and skin

Millet:
supports production of mood-boosting serotonin

Mint:
eases indigestion, promotes detox

Miso:
supports a healthy microbiome

Mulberry:
defends against aging damage, supports healthy hair and nails

Nettle:
strengthens skin and hair

Nutmeg:
supports restful beauty sleep

Nutritional Yeast:
supports healthy hair, skin, and nails

Oats (gluten-free):
supports healthy hair and hair color

Okra:
steadies blood sugar, feeds healthy digestive bacteria

Olive Oil:
defends against UV damage

Olives:
support production of antiaging glutathione

Onion:
blocks wrinkle formation, detoxifies

Orange:
defends against aging damage, reduces the skin's sensitivity to light

Oregano:
antiaging, boosts immune health

Papaya:
defends against sun damage

Parsley:
detoxifies, supports healthy hair and nails

Parsnip:
boosts immune health, supports collagen production

Peach:
maintains glowing skin

Pear:
detoxifies

Peas:
support nervous system function and digestion

Pecans:
promote clear skin, boost immunity

Pepper:
boosts collagen production, reduces inflammation

Pickles (brined):
support a healthy microbiome

Pineapple:
supports healthy hair color and a flat belly

Pistachios:
prevent dry skin

Plum:
preserves collagen and skin firmness

Pomegranate:
maintains healthy collagen, boosts blood flow to skin

Popcorn:
promotes healthy elimination

Potato:
supports healthy hair and hair color

Pumpkin:
heals skin, protects eyes from aging damage

Pumpkin Seeds:
support clear skin and a calm mood

Quinoa:
aids in cell growth and repair

Radish:
builds strong bones and connective tissue

Raspberries:
strengthen hair and nails

Red Cabbage:
builds collagen, strengthens hair and nails

Rhubarb:
defends against sun damage

Romaine Lettuce:
supports smooth skin

Rooibos Tea:
reduces allergies and
defends against UVB
damage

Rosehips:
defend against aging
damage, support
healthy collagen

Rosemary:
boosts mood and
memory

Rutabaga:
reduces redness and
UV damage

Sage:
supports healthy diges-
tion and a flat belly

Sardines:
reduce inflammation

Sauerkraut (raw):
supports a healthy
microbiome

Scallion:
protects eye health
and collagen

Sea Vegetables:
regulate metabolism,
support hormonal
health

Shiitake Mushrooms:
maintain skin elasticity,
support immune health

Spinach:
supports cell renewal
and repair

Sprouts:
boost nutrient
absorption

Stevia:
adds sweetness without
a blood sugar spike

Strawberries:
boost collagen
production

Sugar Snap Peas:
defend against free
radical damage

Sunflower Seeds:
support healthy skin
and scalp

Sweet Potato:
repairs and
smoothes skin

Tahini:
supports clear skin

Teff:
supports cell repair
and energy

Tempeh:
supplies building blocks
of beauty

Thyme:
defends against aging and inflammation

Tomato:
prevents UV damage

Tulsi Tea:
supports a healthy stress response and hormone balance

Turmeric:
reduces inflammation, speeds up healing, relieves pain

Turnip:
reduces redness and UV damage

Walnuts:
support healthy skin and scalp, boost blood flow to skin

Watercress:
defends against and repairs DNA damage

Watermelon:
prevents sun damage, supports antiaging hormone production

White Tea:
defends against the breakdown of collagen and elastin

Wild Rice:
supplies building blocks of beauty

Wild Salmon:
reduces inflammation, supplies building blocks of beauty

Zucchini:
calms nervous function

THE EAT PRETTY PLATE

Whether you're cooking at home, ordering from a restaurant menu, or helping yourself at a party buffet, you'll pack the most beauty benefits onto your plate if you know what to look for in every bite. Quite often I find that beautifying foods possess the same features we admire in the people we consider to be beautiful—freshness, energy, vibrancy. I've also found that beautifying foods share a few very distinctive qualities, listed below. Remember these qualities, and you'll always be able to figure out which foods to pile on and which to pass by.

The acronym **CRAFTS** stands for Colorful, Rich in nutrients, Anti-inflammatory, Fresh, Tailored, and Seasonal. Here's what each of those qualities refers to—and why each one is a beauty must-have:

Colorful. The vibrant natural hues in your food—think purple cabbage, red peppers, and yellow tomatoes—are signs of the powerful phytochemicals (beneficial chemical compounds found in plant foods) contained therein. Phytochemicals (including astaxanthin, sulforaphane, quercetin, and dozens of others) vary widely in their beautifying duties, so instead of trying to memorize them all, just know two things: Phytochemicals are fabulous for your beauty and body, and you should eat as many different kinds (colors) as you can. Some of my favorite phytochemicals—found in foods such as sweet potatoes, berries, and watercress—protect against UV damage, increase skin elasticity, and block wrinkle formation.

Rich in nutrients. The key to getting the most beautifying power out of every morsel of your meal is nutrient density. Take a handful of kale, which delivers over 200 percent of your daily vitamin A needs (a mere 30 calories), or one yellow pepper, with about 600 percent of your vitamin C (just 50 calories). Focus on beauty nutrition first, and you will effortlessly choose foods that fill you up and deliver major nutritional benefits without a need to worry about calories—because you're making every calorie count for so much more. Your body responds to the increased nutrient density of these foods by feeling more satisfied with less. Remember: The less space that low-nutrient foods (think processed foods and sugary sweets) take up on your plate, the more room you have for the foods packed with nutrients that make you glow, energize you, and keep you looking and feeling youthful.

Anti-inflammatory. Inflammation—the body's protective response to infection, irritation, or harm—is bad news for beauty. Not only does chronic, uncontrolled inflammation boost your risk for all kinds of disease, it's a contributing factor in blemishes, premature wrinkles, redness, skin sensitivity, and unwanted weight gain—a huge portion of the beauty pitfalls you're working hard to avoid. Fill your plate with anti-inflammatory foods (such as ginger, wild salmon, and broccoli) and boost beauty from the inside out.

Fresh. We all know fresh is best, right? Too bad it's hard to keep that in mind when you're hungry and reaching for the first convenience food in sight. Packaged, processed, charred, and overcooked foods just don't contain as much living beauty fuel for your body, and at times they even speed up the aging process. So forget the foods designed to stay fresh forever in your cabinet and make room for something just picked, newly ripened, raw or lightly cooked, and, yes, perishable. Your body will thank you.

Tailored. Here's the reason that your optimally beautifying plate looks different from that of your best friend: You are a unique being, with very individual needs. Beauty nutrition is not always one size fits all. You absolutely MUST reflect on the ways that your diet affects your body to know which specific foods enable you to look and feel your best long term.

Seasonal. As you read in the previous section, shifting the foods that you eat and your style of eating with the seasons is the key to targeting your beauty needs head-on. Take note of what's available around you each season, and reach for those foods first.

Filling the Eat Pretty Plate

Now you know what qualities to look for in the foods you put on your plate—what about quantity? The following illustration shows you how to mix up the different categories of foods on your plate for a well-rounded beautifying meal. I recommend that you fill the majority of your plate with veggies and always include some protein and/or healthy fat for beauty nutrition and blood sugar balance. The following illustration includes a few examples of beautifying foods in each category. Remember to tailor your meals, and your particular choices, according to your individual needs.

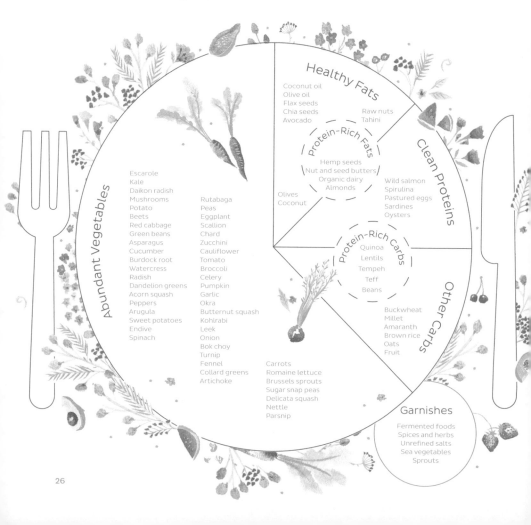

Healthy Fats
Coconut oil
Olive oil
Flax seeds
Chia seeds
Avocado
Raw nuts
Tahini

Protein-Rich Fats
Hemp seeds
Nut and seed butters
Organic dairy
Almonds
Olives
Coconut

Clean Proteins
Wild salmon
Spirulina
Pastured eggs
Sardines
Oysters

Abundant Vegetables
Escarole
Kale
Daikon radish
Mushrooms
Potato
Beets
Red cabbage
Green beans
Asparagus
Cucumber
Burdock root
Watercress
Radish
Dandelion greens
Acorn squash
Peppers
Arugula
Sweet potatoes
Endive
Spinach
Rutabaga
Peas
Eggplant
Scallion
Chard
Zucchini
Cauliflower
Tomato
Broccoli
Celery
Pumpkin
Garlic
Okra
Butternut squash
Kohlrabi
Leek
Onion
Bok choy
Turnip
Fennel
Collard greens
Artichoke
Carrots
Romaine lettuce
Brussels sprouts
Sugar snap peas
Delicata squash
Nettle
Parsnip

Protein-Rich Carbs
Quinoa
Lentils
Tempeh
Teff
Beans

Other Carbs
Buckwheat
Millet
Amaranth
Brown rice
Oats
Fruit

Garnishes
Fermented foods
Spices and herbs
Unrefined salts
Sea vegetables
Sprouts

Portions

A general note about portions: when you're choosing foods that are packed with beauty nutrition, you can ease up on limitations around quantity, and start to listen to your body when it comes to portion sizes. Get used to feeling satisfied and satiated at the end of every meal, both physically and mentally since you're not depriving yourself, but also practice eating until you're just about 80 percent full. I know it's hard, but eating until you're overly stuffed means that you won't truly enjoy, and you might even regret, that last bite or two. Leftovers are bonuses (and make the best next-day breakfasts), so save a little for later! When you reach the point of feeling deeply satisfied with your meals, you break the old pattern of eating, only to want something else 30 minutes later.

Meal Timing

When it comes to eating for beauty, timing is a big consideration. To set up your body for steady energy and blood sugar balance all day long, it helps to eat meals at regular intervals and to avoid long stretches of starvation. If you know you'll be going a long time without a meal, pack a protein-rich snack! Don't skip breakfast, and don't wait until you're cranky and cloudy-headed (a sure sign of low blood sugar) to think about your next meal. Giving your body time to rest and digest between meals and truly savoring and experiencing your food at mealtimes sounds basic, but can be tough to implement. If you can do it, you'll see and feel major beauty benefits!

GROCERY LISTS FOR BEAUTY GOALS

What's your top beauty goal? Whether you're aiming for an energy boost or a clear complexion from the inside out, these grocery lists help you pinpoint the foods that directly support your efforts. Set the goal to include these foods regularly in your colorful, seasonal meals.

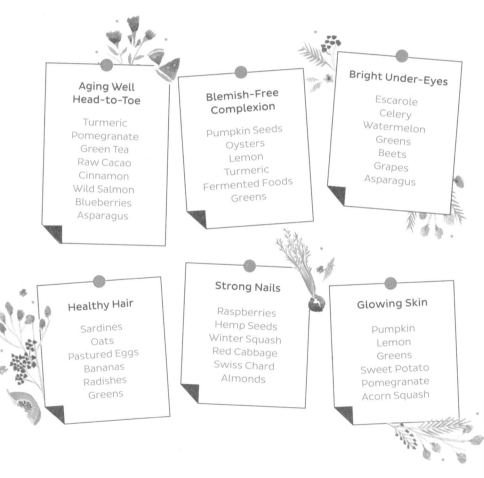

Aging Well Head-to-Toe

Turmeric
Pomegranate
Green Tea
Raw Cacao
Cinnamon
Wild Salmon
Blueberries
Asparagus

Blemish-Free Complexion

Pumpkin Seeds
Oysters
Lemon
Turmeric
Fermented Foods
Greens

Bright Under-Eyes

Escarole
Celery
Watermelon
Greens
Beets
Grapes
Asparagus

Healthy Hair

Sardines
Oats
Pastured Eggs
Bananas
Radishes
Greens

Strong Nails

Raspberries
Hemp Seeds
Winter Squash
Red Cabbage
Swiss Chard
Almonds

Glowing Skin

Pumpkin
Lemon
Greens
Sweet Potato
Pomegranate
Acorn Squash

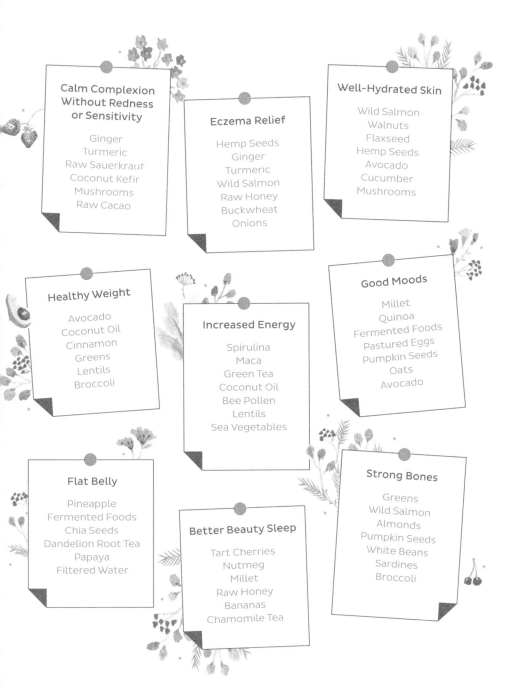

Calm Complexion Without Redness or Sensitivity

Ginger
Turmeric
Raw Sauerkraut
Coconut Kefir
Mushrooms
Raw Cacao

Eczema Relief

Hemp Seeds
Ginger
Turmeric
Wild Salmon
Raw Honey
Buckwheat
Onions

Well-Hydrated Skin

Wild Salmon
Walnuts
Flaxseed
Hemp Seeds
Avocado
Cucumber
Mushrooms

Healthy Weight

Avocado
Coconut Oil
Cinnamon
Greens
Lentils
Broccoli

Increased Energy

Spirulina
Maca
Green Tea
Coconut Oil
Bee Pollen
Lentils
Sea Vegetables

Good Moods

Millet
Quinoa
Fermented Foods
Pastured Eggs
Pumpkin Seeds
Oats
Avocado

Flat Belly

Pineapple
Fermented Foods
Chia Seeds
Dandelion Root Tea
Papaya
Filtered Water

Better Beauty Sleep

Tart Cherries
Nutmeg
Millet
Raw Honey
Bananas
Chamomile Tea

Strong Bones

Greens
Wild Salmon
Almonds
Pumpkin Seeds
White Beans
Sardines
Broccoli

AN IDEAL BEAUTIFYING DAY

Let's all agree right now—perfection does not exist. There's no need to strive for a perfect ideal when we establish that we're all unique. Recall that your beautifying plate looks slightly different from mine, and from the plate of your sister or best friend. The same goes for your daily routine. Embrace that uniqueness. Seize the chance to get to know your body better and adjust your routine based on your personal needs.

That said, while it's pointless to aim for cookie-cutter models of perfection, there are some beautifying components of a daily routine that benefit almost every one of us. What are they? And what is an "ideal beautifying day"? Ahead, you'll find the template for a 24-hour routine packed with beautifying practices and daily essentials to support your mind, body, and beauty. Adjust it, rearrange it, and add to it to meet your needs. But keep the self-nourishing spirit of the day intact, and consider adopting its key elements. Small daily investments in your beauty return to you in the forms of abundant energy, calm, focus, and a radiant glow. In part 3, you'll journal about these investments in yourself as you work toward making every day an ideal beautifying day.

Remember: All day, you can find elements of beauty in whatever you're doing.

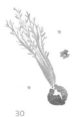

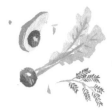

Waking Up

Whether your body awakens on its own or you open your eyes to the sound of an alarm, you greet the day feeling refreshed (because your hormones are in balance and you've met your quota for restful beauty sleep), without snoozing an alarm four times in succession. Instead of grabbing your smartphone or bolting out of bed, you lie under the covers for a moment and breathe in deeply, feeling your abdomen rise and fall. You feel the weight of your body, stretch gently to reawaken it, and think about one exciting or positive thing that could happen today, without fast-forwarding to moments that could be stressful or difficult. Do this, and you set the stage for calm and focus (rather than skyrocketing stress hormones) before your feet even hit the floor.

You head to the kitchen for some warm lemon water (add fresh ginger and/or turmeric for extra beauty points). You take a few quiet moments to sip your beauty drink while you map out the day ahead, set intentions that will help you meet your beauty and health (or other) goals, and reflect with gratitude on the day to come. What are you grateful for right now, before this day has even begun? Gratitude breeds joy and contentment—two healthy, antiaging emotions that seriously deepen your glow!

Morning

After you've settled in and taken time to set your beautifying day into motion, you allow technology into your morning—check email, voicemail, social media . . . anything you need to prepare for the tasks ahead.

Regardless of what your unique morning routine looks like, eat an energizing, beautifying breakfast that includes protein and/or healthy fat (and ideally some veggies as well). Breakfast sets the stage for the way you will think, feel, perform, and, yes, eat for the entire day. For this reason, I see it as the most important meal to get right. Make it a priority to eat breakfast within 90 minutes of waking for optimal blood sugar stability. Forget sources of refined carbs and sugar like pastries, donuts, most cereals, and yogurts. Even forego the juice, unless you're going for veggie juice, and you're pairing it with other protein and healthy fat sources. Don't feel hungry? Sometimes stress can dull your hunger signals, so be sure to eat something— however small—that contains protein and/or healthy fat. Try avocado toast or a light smoothie with a protein source like hemp seeds.

Now that you're focused, fueled, and have taken some time for self-care, get going. This would be a great time for exercise—a quick morning yoga session, jog, walk, or whatever energizes you and gets you moving without adding extra stress into your day. This time is also ideal to practice meditation, a kind of strength-training session for your body's calm and focus muscles. If you don't have time for these essentials now, try to make time later in your day. The middle of the morning is an ideal time to have a beautifying snack, especially if you had an early breakfast and will wait a long stretch before lunch. Favorite beauty-friendly snacks include chia pudding, raw trail mix, hummus and veggies, roasted chickpeas, or a hard-boiled egg.

Mid-Day

Your digestion is strong mid-day, so make lunch a complete, nourishing beauty meal. About fifteen minutes before you sit down to eat, drink a glass of water to hydrate your digestive tract and prepare for optimal digestion. Take another moment to breathe deeply (notice a pattern here?) before you pick up your fork, and eat slowly and mindfully, chewing well. Lunch is a great time to convene with friends or colleagues, since person-to-person connection is also an important part of your day!

Afternoon

Break for a mid-afternoon snack if you tend to eat a late dinner. Again, make it nutrient-dense, and be sure it includes some protein and/or healthy fat to support energy and hormone balance. In addition to your snack, give yourself time to pause and be present in your day.

Evening

Have a relaxed dinner when you feel ready and you've have had time to prepare (or seek out) a nourishing meal. Complex carbs like sweet potatoes, lentils, and quinoa are wonderful to include in your dinner since they support the production of calming serotonin that helps you sleep well. Overall, try not to eat too late: You want to free up energy to repair and cleanse your body during the night, rather than using precious, restorative energy for digestion.

Before Bed

Wind down with a cup of calming tea or magnesium drink, and/or take a muscle-relaxing Epsom salt soak in the evening. Curl up in bed in your pj's and sleep soundly all night. When you stay up too late, your body often gets a second wind caused by a surge of cortisol that can make it hard to fall asleep and sleep well, whenever you do eventually settle down to rest. You should base your daily sleep patterns on your body's own needs; most of us feel best with between 7 and 9 hours of rest each night.

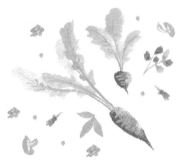

The Daily Essentials: Beauty Nutrition & Self-Care

Adding these daily habits (as many as you can fit!) to your routine is a major leap toward more vibrant health and radiant beauty overall. These essentials make the most significant impact in the lives of my clients who seek a glowing complexion, shiny hair, stronger nails, increased energy, and a slimmer waistline. Altogether, they guide you to a truly beautifying lifestyle.

BEAUTY NUTRITION

Incorporate these nutritional elements into your routine to nourish your beauty from the inside.

Warm lemon water

Squeeze the juice of half a lemon into a mug, top with warm water (which is the temperature level that best supports morning elimination), and sip as you start your day for detoxification, internal cleansing, optimal digestion, alkalinity, and a collagen and immunity boost. For extra antioxidant, anti-inflammatory value, add fresh or ground ginger and/or turmeric.

One or more servings of greens

Aim to eat a varied spectrum of foods and colors each day, but always be certain that you include plenty of greens. Their detoxifying, healing, skin-clearing properties are critical for optimal beauty.

Seasonal fruits and vegetables

When you can, opt for fresh, seasonal foods, which often offer the most concentrated, and targeted, beauty nutrition.

Protein and/or healthy fat at each meal

Blood sugar stability is one of the secrets to gorgeous skin, energy, reaching and maintaining an ideal weight, and hormone balance, as well as slowing the aging process. At each meal, remember to include beautifying proteins and/or healthy fats when you assemble your plate.

Probiotics and/or fermented foods

To achieve your healthiest, most beautiful glow, make digestive support a priority. Probiotic supplements are great everyday insurance for better digestion, but small daily servings of fermented foods will take things to the next level with even more gut-strengthening benefits.

Complete, mindful chewing at snack and mealtime

Don't miss the chance to further support strong digestion and assimilation of your beauty foods and their powerful nutrients while you chew each bite. Compared to eating your greens, chewing may seem like an insignificant contribution to your beauty. But when done mindfully, it can make a big overall impact on your digestive processes.

Fresh herbs and spices

One of the easiest—and most delicious—ways to add instant antioxidant, antiaging, and beautifying power to your current meals is to incorporate ample herbs and spices. Get familiar with your spice rack; experiment with new seasonings in your recipes; plant an herb garden and harvest from it daily. The phytochemicals in these flavorful foods deliver potent beauty benefits even in small doses.

Regular meal intervals

Spacing out your meals supports optimal blood sugar balance and digestion, and ensures that you don't face a sudden energy slump during the day. It's worth the extra attention to plan ahead for regularly spaced meals and healthy snacks when you need them.

Frequent hydration

Your skin is 70 percent water, and your body requires this essential fluid to perform some of its most critical beauty functions, like digestion, nutrient absorption, metabolism, and waste removal. Plus, when you're low on water, your skin loses its radiant glow.

Supplements, if applicable

If you take supplements—such as a multivitamin, fish oil, or vitamin D— for extra beauty nutrients or other nutritional support, take them at a regular time so you won't forget them in your busy day.

SELF-CARE

Set aside regular time for these habits to discover a more balanced and beautifying existence.

Meditation and/or quiet time

Sitting quietly and releasing all conscious thoughts from your mind—which can be attempted by concentrating solely on each inhale and exhale and letting go of every worry, question, and wandering thought as it enters your mind—for just five or ten minutes has profound benefits for your stress levels, hormone balance, focus, calm, and beauty. As an alternative, simply give yourself quiet time away from the sensory stimulation of the world.

Deep breathing

We spend much of the day rushing from task to task while taking short, shallow breaths. Breathing is an important source of detoxification and waste removal for the body, and deep, abdominal breaths trigger a relaxation response that can quickly lower stress levels. Deep breaths are also a reminder to be present in all that you do.

Physical activity

Moving your body increases circulation of beauty nutrients and brings an incomparable glow to your complexion. Focus on the feeling—rather than the calorie burn—that you get from exercise to figure out what suits you best. And when in doubt, just play!

Connection with friends or family

Regular social interactions have incredibly impactful benefits for health, longevity, and antiaging. (Of course, opt for positive, stress-free interactions whenever you can!) We're all busy, but don't underestimate the power of connecting with a friend to enhance something as beautifying as deep breathing or hormone balance, thanks to the lower stress hormones and activation of the parasympathetic nervous system that come from regular supportive connection.

De-stressing activity

Stress has such a constant presence in our modern lives that we need deliberate, daily time set aside to counteract its aging effects. Your stress-lowering moments can come in the form of exercise, social interaction, self-love, meditation, journaling, or any of the other beautifying habits that you're following daily.

Self-love
The beautifying powers of daily self-love can't be overstated. Taking time to do something nice for yourself every day—something totally separate from your daily pampering meals—is a tiny way to profoundly increase your overall happiness with your self and your life. Ask yourself what you need each day, and respond accordingly. Buy fresh flowers, give yourself a mini-facial, take time out to read a book—choose anything that makes you feel happy and cared for.

Beauty sleep
Sleep is free repair and antiaging for your entire body. Turn off the TV, put down your phone, and make time for it tonight.

Affirmations
"I am strong." "I am naturally beautiful." "I am full of creative energy." What are the affirming words you need to reinforce your beauty and look and feel your best today? There is power in thinking and saying daily affirmations.

Intentions
Take a few minutes each morning to set healthy, beautifying intentions for the day ahead, and you'll stay more committed to your goals. A daily intention can be as simple as "I will eat more colorful veggies today," or as complex as "I will be present and mindful in all that I do today." Think of an intention as a mini-challenge for your body to fulfill, one that supports you in all things beautiful.

Gratitude
Studies show that gratitude increases happiness, reduces depression and regret, and even supports better beauty sleep and stronger immunity. I maintain that it also makes you glow. What are you grateful for in this beautiful life?

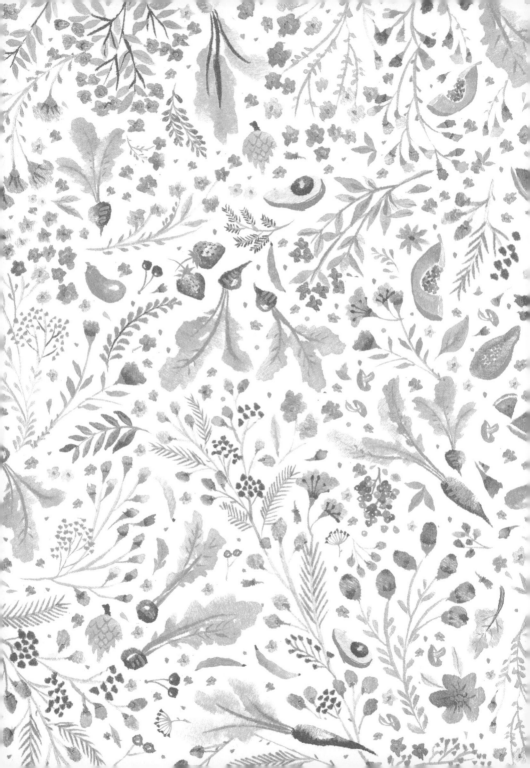

PART 2

CHARTING A BEAUTIFUL LIFE

WHEN I WORK WITH CLIENTS ONE ON ONE, our greatest tool for change is reflection. We look for patterns: foods that may be causing negative reactions in the body, or particular mind-sets or beliefs that could be holding back a healthy new habit. Beyond seeing amazing transformations happen, the opportunity to reflect and create moments of true self-discovery simply from looking at everyday habits is my favorite part of health coaching. When else do we take the opportunity to look closely at ourselves, with the added goal of a beauty tune-up?

When it comes to beauty, our most profound discovery is often the deep connection between nutrition and the way we look and feel. Whether you learned about that connection years ago, or it's something you're considering right now for the first time, it's incredibly motivating to recognize the immense power you have to shape your beauty every single day. The Q&As, lists, and trackers in the pages ahead will encourage you to take control of that power and play an active role in the way you look and feel. It's not enough to just grab a product off a store shelf and think it will affect the changes you're seeking. This is the moment to get involved, be inspired, and record the exciting shifts that are happening in the way you look and feel!

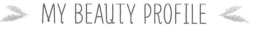

MY BEAUTY PROFILE

Grab a pen or pencil and explore your individual beauty story. Reflect on the role that beauty plays in your life, rate the areas of your beauty and health that may need the most attention, and consider the characteristics you love most about your unique body.

Age: 27

Your three favorite physical traits:

1 My cheekbones
2 My eyelashes
3 My thighs

Your three favorite personality traits:

1 My sense of humour
2 My ability to socialize
3 My work ethic

List any supplements you're currently taking.

Iron - on + off

On a scale of 1 (needs work) to 5 (optimal), rate the current health of your . . . (circle one):

Skin	1 2 ③ 4 5
Hair	1 2 3 ④ 5
Nails	① 2 3 4 5
Energy	1 ② 3 4 5
Weight	1 ② 3 4 5
Moods	1 ② 3 4 5
Resilience to stress	1 ② 3 4 5

When was the last time you looked and felt your best? Describe that feeling and moment.

when I felt thinner, hair was full + lusious. felt sexy in my own skin. Looked at my body in the mirror, and liked what I saw.

What do you love most about your current diet?	What would you most like to change about your current diet?
when I cook for myself. It's healthy.	The amount of food I eat.

List any foods you regularly crave.	How many hours of sleep do you need each night?	How often do you get that many hours of sleep?
Burgers, cheese, bread, pasta.	8	Most nights.

List any known allergies or sensitivities to food.	Have you ever been diagnosed with a skin condition (acne, rosacea, eczema, etc.)? If so, what treatment did you receive?
None - that I know of.	NO.

List any known allergies or sensitivities to ingredients in personal care products.	
I think I have general sensitive skin.	

What's your favorite step in your current beauty routine?	What's your least favorite step in your current beauty routine?
Curling my hair.	All of it.

Do you have any digestive health concerns? If so, list them.	Do you have any hormonal health concerns? If so, list them.
NO.	NO.

SEASONAL BEAUTY FOODS CHECKLIST

How many have you tried? Check off all the seasonal beauty foods you've included in your diet to date. The unchecked boxes will illuminate the beauty foods you may want to taste next. Challenge yourself to check all the boxes by the year's end! (Beauty bonus: Refer to page 16 [Beauty Foods from A to Z] to see the beauty benefits you're inviting into your life by sampling these foods.)

SPRING

- ☐ Artichoke
- ☒ Arugula
- ☒ Asparagus
- ☒ Bok Choy
- ☐ Coconut
- ☐ Dandelion Greens
- ☐ Endive
- ☒ Garlic

- ☒ Green Beans
- ☒ Lemon
- ☒ Lime
- ☐ Nettle
- ☐ Peas
- ☐ Radish
- ☐ Rhubarb
- ☒ Romaine Lettuce

- ☒ Scallion
- ☒ Spinach
- ☒ Sprouts
- ☒ Strawberries
- ☐ Sugar Snap Peas
- ☐ Watercress

SUMMER

- ☒ Apricots
- ☒ Blackberries
- ☒ Blueberries
- ☒ Cantaloupe
- ☒ Celery
- ☒ Cherries
- ☐ Collard Greens

- ☒ Cucumber
- ☒ Eggplant
- ☐ Mulberry
- ☐ Okra
- ☐ Papaya
- ☒ Peach
- ☒ Pepper

- ☒ Pineapple
- ☒ Plum
- ☒ Raspberries
- ☒ Tomato
- ☒ Watermelon
- ☒ Zucchini

AUTUMN

- ☐ Acorn Squash
- ☒ Apple
- ☒ Broccoli
- ☐ Burdock Root
- ☐ Butternut Squash
- ☐ Chard
- ☒ Cranberries

- ☒ Daikon Radish
- ☐ Delicata Squash
- ☐ Escarole
- ☐ Figs
- ☒ Grapes
- ☐ Kohlrabi
- ☒ Leek

- ☒ Pear
- ☐ Pumpkin
- ☒ Red Cabbage
- ☐ Rosehips
- ☐ Rutabaga
- ☒ Shiitake Mushroom
- ☐ Sweet Potato

WINTER

- ☒ Avocado
- ☒ Banana
- ☐ Beets
- ☒ Brussels Sprouts
- ☒ Carrot
- ☒ Cauliflower

- ☐ Fennel
- ☐ Grapefruit
- ☒ Kale
- ☒ Kiwi
- ☒ Onion
- ☒ Orange

- ☐ Parsnip
- ☐ Pomegranate
- ☒ Potato
- ☐ Turnip

FOODS IN YOUR YEAR-ROUND PANTRY

- [x] Almond Milk
- [x] Almonds
- [ ] Amaranth
- [x] Apple Cider Vinegar
- [ ] Beans
- [ ] Bee Pollen
- [ ] Blackstrap Molasses
- [ ] Brazil Nuts
- [ ] Buckwheat
- [ ] Cacao
- [x] Cashews
- [x] Chia Seeds
- [ ] Chickpeas
- [ ] Coconut Milk
- [ ] Coconut Oil
- [x] Dates
- [x] Flaxseed
- [ ] Goji Berries
- [ ] Hemp Seeds
- [x] Honey (raw)
- [ ] Kimchi
- [x] Lentils
- [ ] Maple Syrup
- [ ] Millet
- [ ] Miso
- [ ] Nutritional Yeast
- [x] Oats (gluten-free)
- [x] Olive Oil
- [x] Olives
- [ ] Pecans
- [x] Pickles (brined)
- [ ] Pistachios
- [ ] Popcorn
- [ ] Pumpkin Seeds
- [x] Quinoa
- [ ] Sardines
- [x] Sauerkraut (raw)
- [ ] Sea Vegetables (nori, dulse, kelp, kombu, spirulina, wakame)
- [ ] Stevia
- [ ] Sunflower Seeds
- [x] Tahini
- [ ] Teff
- [ ] Tempeh
- [ ] Walnuts
- [x] Wild Rice
- [x] Wild Salmon

HERBS AND SPICES

- [x] Basil
- [x] Black Pepper
- [ ] Cardamom
- [ ] Cayenne
- [ ] Chives
- [ ] ~~Cilantro~~
- [ ] Cinnamon
- [ ] Cloves
- [ ] Cumin
- [x] Dill
- [ ] Fennel Seeds
- [x] Ginger
- [ ] Mint
- [ ] Nutmeg
- [x] Oregano
- [x] Parsley
- [x] Rosemary
- [ ] Sage
- [x] Thyme
- [ ] Turmeric

TEAS

- [x] Chamomile
- [ ] Dandelion Root
- [x] Ginger
- [x] Green
- [ ] Rooibos
- [ ] Tulsi
- [x] White

MY BEAUTY GOALS

List your ongoing beauty goals on the following chart to keep track of the ways you boost your beauty and health over hours, days, months, and years. Simple yet powerful beauty-boosting goals include cooking a healthy new meal every day this week, or trying five new beauty foods this month, while more intensive beauty goals might be initiating a daily ten-minute meditation session, or scheduling a regular get-together with friends.

Start by entering your goal on the left side of this chart, along with the current date, and the status of your goal. Then, in the weeks ahead, turn back to these pages and use the Check-in box to record your progress—or, if you've already achieved the goal, skip directly to the Goal Met box to check it off and record your results.

Goal	Current Status	Check-in Status
Meditate everyday for 15-30 min.	Start Date: Jan. 21	Date:
Wash face at the end of everyday + Shower body everyother day	Start Date:	Date:
Try new recipe once a week	Start Date:	Date:
Exercise 2 times a week at least	Start Date:	Date:

Goal Met	Notes
Date:	
Results:	
Date:	
Results:	
Date:	
Results:	
Date:	
Results:	

FOOD RELATIONSHIP Q&A

There's no denying it: Our relationships with food are complicated. Emotions, memories, outside pressures, and cravings all interfere with our efforts to eat for beauty and health. This section invites you to reflect on your current relationship with food, identify complicating factors, and improve the role food plays in your life.

What challenges prevent you from eating well on an average day?	How can you tackle these challenges?
Cravings, lack of energy to cook, temptations	Plan ahead, bring snacks

On a scale of 1 (needs work) to 5 (optimal), rate your current ability to . . . (circle one):

	1	2	3	4	5
Cook beautifying meals at home	1	2	③	4	5
Pack healthy meals and snacks to take with you	1	②	3	4	5
Eat regularly spaced meals	1	②	3	4	5
Create a balanced, Eat Pretty plate	1	2	3	④	5
Navigate the grocery store to find beauty foods	1	2	3	④	5
Eat calmly, without stress	1	②	3	4	5
Select and eat adequate portions	1	②	3	4	5
Recognize and interpret your response to foods	1	②	3	4	5
Pause, breathe, and reflect in between bites	①	2	3	4	5
Chew each bite thoroughly	①	2	3	4	5
Feel nourished and satisfied after eating	1	②	3	4	5

Describe a time when you noticed that food positively impacted your beauty.	Describe a time when you noticed that food negatively impacted your beauty.
	After eating large amount of food feeling sluggish and bloated.

List three foods that make you feel guilty after eating them.	In what situations would you be able to enjoy them, guilt-free?
• Fries • Mcdonalds • Ice Cream	• Socially • After drinking

List three foods that make you feel energized.	How can you incorporate more of these foods into your diet?
• Broccoli, • Carrots • Salmon	• have them in my fridge chopped or cooked. • make time for food prep

List three foods that make you feel pampered.	How can you incorporate more of these foods into your diet?

List three foods that make you feel satisfied.	How can you incorporate more of these foods into your diet?

What would you like to change or improve about your current relationship with food?

RECIPES TO TRY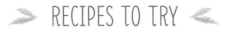

Use this section to record recipes that you'd like to try—or ones you've created. Look out for recipes that help you nourish yourself and your loved ones in a healthy way, recipes for easy-prep meals, and recipes that incorporate your favorite beauty foods.

Recipe Name

Ingredients	Preparation Instructions

Recipe Name

Ingredients	Preparation Instructions

Recipe Name

Ingredients	Preparation Instructions

THE EAT PRETTY PANTRY: TO-DO LIST

Shopping for fresh foods is easy enough; the challenge arises when you return to your kitchen and find that you're missing the key ingredients you need to transform these foods into a satisfying meal. Build an Eat Pretty pantry to ensure that you always have the best, most beautifying ingredients on hand to pair with fresh beauty foods. The suggested swaps, eliminations, and additions outlined in this section highlight key pantry staples that enable you to cook beautifying daily meals using the just-picked, seasonal foods you bring home from the market. Follow these steps to a more beautiful cooking experience.

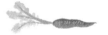

To Do: Reduce or Eliminate Beauty Betrayers

Are you staring into crowded cabinets, wondering which foods and items to weed out in the name of beauty? This quick-reference list can help. These are the Beauty Betrayers—the foods that are not doing any favors for your skin, hair, nails, weight, energy, and mood (learn more on page 12). Remove these food categories from your diet and your pantry as often as you are able. As you make this commitment—throwing them out as necessary, or resolving to reduce your intake—check the box and prepare to glow.

☐ Alcohol
☐ Caffeine
☐ Canned foods with BPA
☐ Dairy
☐ Fried Foods
☐ Gluten

☐ Grilled and Overcooked Foods
☐ Meats (conventional)
☐ Pesticide-Sprayed Produce
☐ Processed Foods
☐ Soda
☐ Sugar

To Do: Toss This, Try That

Some items in your pantry may fall into the Beauty Betrayer category while others might simply lack significant beauty benefits. Many of these foods can be replaced with a substitute—one that's just as delicious, and better for your beauty overall. I promise, many of these swaps are effortless! Refer to the lists below for guidance on what to toss and what to try as a replacement. As you complete each swap, check the corresponding boxes and appreciate how you're supercharging the beauty nutrition in your cabinets!

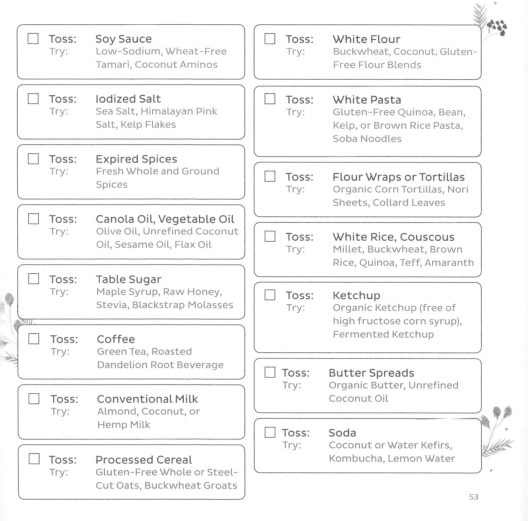

☐ Toss: **Soy Sauce**
　 Try: Low-Sodium, Wheat-Free Tamari, Coconut Aminos

☐ Toss: **Iodized Salt**
　 Try: Sea Salt, Himalayan Pink Salt, Kelp Flakes

☐ Toss: **Expired Spices**
　 Try: Fresh Whole and Ground Spices

☐ Toss: **Canola Oil, Vegetable Oil**
　 Try: Olive Oil, Unrefined Coconut Oil, Sesame Oil, Flax Oil

☐ Toss: **Table Sugar**
　 Try: Maple Syrup, Raw Honey, Stevia, Blackstrap Molasses

☐ Toss: **Coffee**
　 Try: Green Tea, Roasted Dandelion Root Beverage

☐ Toss: **Conventional Milk**
　 Try: Almond, Coconut, or Hemp Milk

☐ Toss: **Processed Cereal**
　 Try: Gluten-Free Whole or Steel-Cut Oats, Buckwheat Groats

☐ Toss: **White Flour**
　 Try: Buckwheat, Coconut, Gluten-Free Flour Blends

☐ Toss: **White Pasta**
　 Try: Gluten-Free Quinoa, Bean, Kelp, or Brown Rice Pasta, Soba Noodles

☐ Toss: **Flour Wraps or Tortillas**
　 Try: Organic Corn Tortillas, Nori Sheets, Collard Leaves

☐ Toss: **White Rice, Couscous**
　 Try: Millet, Buckwheat, Brown Rice, Quinoa, Teff, Amaranth

☐ Toss: **Ketchup**
　 Try: Organic Ketchup (free of high fructose corn syrup), Fermented Ketchup

☐ Toss: **Butter Spreads**
　 Try: Organic Butter, Unrefined Coconut Oil

☐ Toss: **Soda**
　 Try: Coconut or Water Kefirs, Kombucha, Lemon Water

To Do: Preserve Beauty Nutrition

Storing your pantry foods properly can help preserve their nutrition—and make sure you get the beauty benefits you're banking on. To preserve flavor and freshness and maintain potent beauty benefits, freeze or refrigerate the following foods, and check each box once the food has been stored optimally.

FREEZE

- ☐ Raw Nuts and Seeds Not in Use
- ☐ Fresh Ginger and Turmeric
- ☐ Gluten-Free Flours

REFRIGERATE

- ☐ Oils
- ☐ Nut Butters
- ☐ Raw Nuts and Seeds in Use
- ☐ Probiotics and Digestive Enzymes
- ☐ Vinegars

To Do: Stock Up on Staples

Some staple foods are so versatile for cooking healthy meals, and so beneficial to your beauty, they deserve a regular place in your cabinets. Stock up on these beauty food staples, checking them off as you go, so you'll always have them on hand to cook a beauty-boosting meal with the addition of fresh produce.

- ☐ Amaranth
- ☐ Buckwheat
- ☐ Black Beans
- ☐ Brown Rice
- ☐ Chickpeas
- ☐ Kidney Beans
- ☐ Lentils

- ☐ Millet
- ☐ Oats (gluten-free)
- ☐ Pinto Beans
- ☐ Quinoa
- ☐ Teff
- ☐ White Beans
- ☐ Wild Rice

SEASONAL BEAUTY CHALLENGES

For everything, there is a season. Take these words to heart as you build your lifestyle of beauty and fill your plate with the foods that best meet your shifting seasonal beauty needs. Here's a season-by-season look at top challenges you can pose to yourself to support the health of your beauty and body. Start with the current season and its respective challenges, and check the box when you've made the commitment. When the next season arrives, commit to its goals, and so on. Using the blank spaces, add your own challenges to inspire your personal dedication to your beauty and health year-round.

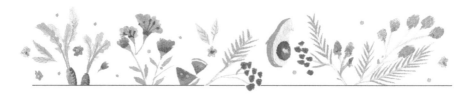

Spring

The energetic potential of spring is palpable. The air smells alive, the sun's rays electrify you, and you enter a period of renewal, detoxification, and lightening that at times can be quite literal. In spring, focus on refreshing your lifestyle, reinventing yourself, awakening your spirit and your connection to the world around you, and making a new commitment to beautifying habits that may have fallen by the wayside over the winter. Fill your plate with greens and other fresh, green foods. Your reward will be glowing skin, shedding excess "winter weight," and increasing your energy levels.

SPRING CHALLENGES
This season, I will . . .

☐ Eat plenty of fresh, alkaline greens and spring foods like asparagus, artichokes, and sprouts.

☐ Embrace foods with a bitter taste (this signals cleansing), like dandelion greens and watercress.

☐ Choose organic produce and toxin-free cosmetics with natural and organic ingredients.

☐ Chew food thoroughly to encourage complete digestion and assimilation.

☐ Dry brush my skin to encourage detoxification and lymphatic drainage.

☐ Eat more lightly cooked or raw foods.

☐ Consider taking probiotics or eating fermented foods daily to encourage strong digestion, healthy weight, and a flat belly.

☐ _____

☐ _____

☐ _____

☐ _____

☐ _____

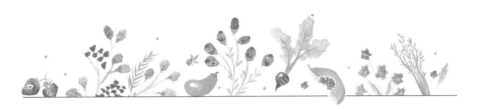

Summer

Summer marks the height of the year's energy, activity, heat, and abundance. It's the season when the senses awaken—on your plate and in the world around you. Let the environment and the fresh foods of the season peak your energy and your desire to keep eating for beauty. Beauty food should be bursting with flavor and hydration this season! There's so much variety and color at the farmers' market, so change the ingredients in your meals as often as possible. Many colorful summer foods help protect your skin from UV damage, cool you, and deepen your skin's natural glow.

SUMMER CHALLENGES

This season, I will . . .

☐ Prioritize hydration with naturally water-rich and bloat-releasing foods like celery, cucumber, coconut water, and pineapple.

☐ Move daily, with the type of exercise that suits me best.

☐ Connect with the outdoors—the sun, the earth, fresh air—and experience nature in its peak season.

☐ Shield my skin with safe sun care and UV-protective summer foods like bell peppers, watermelon, tomatoes, and papaya.

☐ Grow fresh food.

☐ Opt for plenty of summer foods that give skin a golden glow, like cantaloupe, apricots, and peaches.

☐ _____

☐ _____

☐ _____

☐ _____

☐ _____

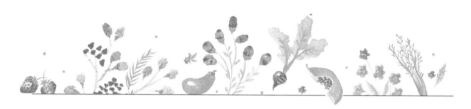

Autumn

Autumn is a transitional season that sometimes mimics summer, and at other times shocks you with wintry chills. Your energy remains high in autumn, so it's an ideal season to be goal-oriented and complete projects. But you're beginning to cool and detoxify your body from the heat and abundance of the summer in preparation for winter rest. When it comes to beauty, autumn is a season of healing and balancing the skin after its exposure to the harsh summer elements, so fill up on the massive harvest of nutrient-dense autumn beauty foods.

AUTUMN CHALLENGES
This season, I will . . .

- [ ] Eat meals that combine raw and cooked foods to reflect this transitional time of the year.
- [ ] Choose nutrient-dense, skin-healing autumn vegetables like squash and pumpkin to repair summer damage.
- [ ] Take advantage of the energy and industriousness of the season to experiment with new foods and recipes.
- [ ] Support detox with fresh, fiber-rich foods and plenty of fluids.
- [ ] Balance mounting work and school schedules with daily meditation.
- [ ] Eliminate one new Beauty Betrayer this autumn, the season of letting go.
- [ ] Opt for root vegetables like beets and sweet potatoes for their natural balancing and grounding effects that also reduce sweet cravings.
- [ ] _____
- [ ] _____
- [ ] _____
- [ ] _____
- [ ] _____

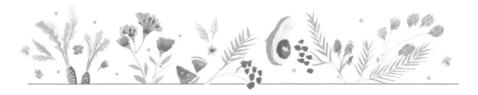

Winter

With shorter days and longer nights, nature gives you permission to slow down this season. Focus on nourishing food, optimal sleep, and calm during the winter months. Take time to move your body and boost your circulation with exercises that keep you fit without exhausting you. Beauty goals of the season include keeping immunity strong, preventing seasonal skin dryness, inflammation, and sensitivity, avoiding unnecessary weight gain from holiday celebrations, and preparing the body for spring rebirth.

WINTER CHALLENGES

This season, I will . . .

- ☒ Rest and recharge my body regularly and fully.
- ☒ Stay in tune with my hunger and fullness, even while celebrating.
- ☒ Take time to prepare more warm, home-cooked meals.
- ☒ Ward off colds and flu with immune-boosting foods like onions, garlic, mushrooms, cruciferous veggies, and citrus fruits.
- ☒ Keep skin hydrated with healthy fats ike avocado and coconut oil, and warm liquids like herbal teas, lemon water, and ginger/turmeric infusions.
- ☒ Add abundant warming, circulation-boosting spices to meals.
- ☐ Exercise more
- ☐ Eat energizing snacks
- ☐
- ☐
- ☐

SELF-LOVE Q&A

Self-love is a powerful force that drives our efforts to eat for beauty and create a beautifying life. This section invites you to reflect on your current capacity for self-love, identify areas of your life that could use more self-love, and explore new ideas for loving yourself more deeply each day.

On a scale of 1 (needs work) to 5 (optimal), how well do you . . . (circle one):

Love yourself unconditionally	1	②	3	4	5
Identify your personal needs	1	2	3	④	5
Respond to those personal needs	1	2	③	4	5
Pamper yourself regularly	1	2	③	4	5
Feel confident in your beauty	1	②	3	4	5
Embrace your body and beauty without judgment	1	②	3	4	5
Trust your inner wisdom and instincts	1	2	3	④	5
Feel committed to your personal happiness	1	2	3	④	5

When did you last indulge in something that made you feel good? What was the indulgence?	Identify one activity that makes you happy that you would like to do more often.
Hot bath with weed and music.	Walking while listening to music.

Identify a situation that causes you to feel negative, or to treat yourself with negativity.

Dating.

What can you do to prevent this negativity the next time you're in this situation?

Trust myself. Move slowly. Spend time with friends.. Meditate. Journal

List three things you love about your body and beauty.	When you're feeling run-down, how do you restore yourself and rebuild your strength?
1 I have a good figure. Big boobs, nice butt.	I sleep Clean Shower Meditate.
2 My hair colour is unique + pretty	
3 I have nice lips + a nice smile	

List three things you can do to reward yourself that don't involve food.	Name three people who boost your self-love and confidence.
1 Smoke weed	1 Karen
2 watch a movie	2 Mama
3	3 Loren

WORDS THAT INSPIRE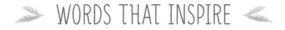

Repeating an affirmation or mantra helps fine-tune your focus and empowers you to strengthen your lifestyle of beauty every day. A few of my favorites are:

I breathe in wellness and exhale stress.
I am strong and resilient.
Happiness builds radiance.
I find unexpected beauty in everyday moments.
My body knows its needs and guides me to them.

Use this space to create your own inspiring sayings, or record those you've heard from friends, mentors, and loved ones, for motivation when you need it most.

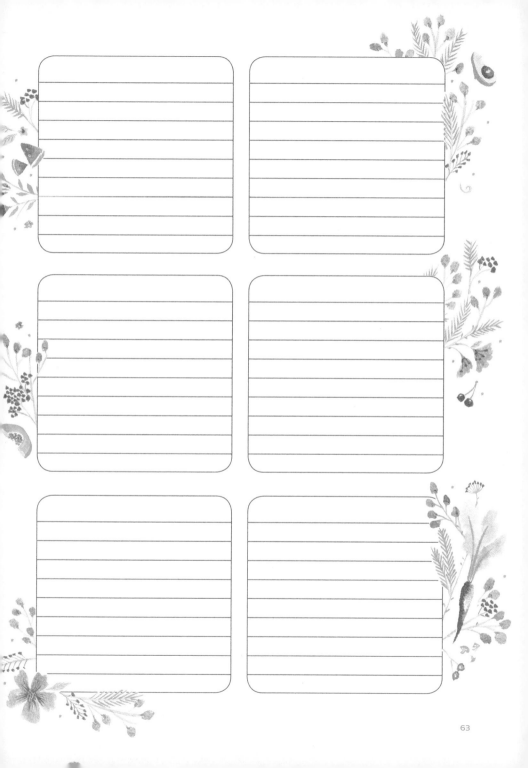

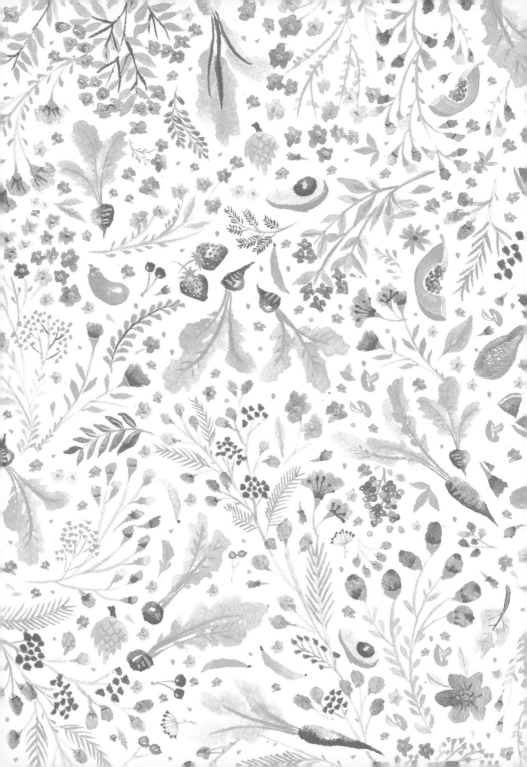

PART 3

40 DAYS OF EAT PRETTY

AT THIS POINT IN YOUR JOURNAL EXPERIENCE, I hope you feel focused and inspired. The following 40 journal entries—each designed to capture a day's worth of meals and self-care activities—help you shift occasional beautifying habits into a transformative routine, and reflect on the ways that your meals influence how you look and feel each day. You can decide when, and how often, to use these journal entries. You might complete all 40 entries over 40 consecutive days, creating your own intensive beauty overhaul. You might fill out one entry every week, spreading out your experience over 40 weeks. Or you might turn to a new entry whenever you feel like reconnecting with your goals and reinforcing your beautifying habits. Every ten entries, you will encounter a check-in section that invites you to pause and look back on your progress over time, identify challenges and successes, and apply that knowledge to the future. Over time, with thought and reflection, you will bring new sides of your beauty and health to light.

DATE:

Current Season:

- ☐ **SPRING**
  the season of detox, renewal, lightening
- ☐ **SUMMER**
  the season of sun defense, hydration, activity
- ☐ **AUTUMN**
  the season of healing, balancing, grounding
- ☒ **WINTER**
  the season of nourishment, rest, preparation

Today's positive affirmation:

I am *strong and beautiful.*

Today I am grateful for:

Karen's love + friendship.

Today's health and beauty goals:

To clear my body, a partner and make warm food.

Beauty Nutrition Essentials I Enjoyed Today:

- ☐ Warm lemon water
- ☐ One or more servings of greens
- ☐ Seasonal fruit and veggies
- ☒ Protein and/or healthy fat at each meal
- ☐ Probiotics and/or fermented food
- ☐ Complete, mindful chewing at snack and mealtimes
- ☐ Fresh herbs and spices
- ☐ Regular meal intervals
- ☐ Frequent hydration (including ___ glasses of water)
- ☐ Supplements, if applicable
- ☐ Other:

Self-Care Essentials I Enjoyed Today:

- ☒ Meditation and/or quiet time
- ☐ Deep breathing
- ☒ Physical activity
- ☒ Connection with friends or family
- ☐ De-stressing activity
- ☒ Self-love
- ☒ Beauty sleep (*2* hours) *nap.*
- ☐ Other:

DAILY FOOD DIARY

Breakfast
What I ate:

Reuben Sandwich

Time 11:00 am | Setting: Granville Island

How I felt after eating:

Not super full.
Tired / lethargic.
But it was so
good.

Lunch
What I ate: Pita, Israeli salad, kugel, shakshuka, kalbose, 1/4 bagel, cheese

Time 3:00 pm | Setting: hone

How I felt after eating:

Satisfied, gassy, tired.

Dinner
What I ate:

Veggie soup
Sausage

Time 8:00 | Setting: hone

How I felt after eating:

Satisfied
gassy

Other
Today's snacks:

grapes

Favorite beauty foods I ate today:

soup
grapes
salad
tomato sauce

When did you look and feel your best today?

Look- Morning
Feel- when @ granville Island

Takeaways from today:

Eat less sausage + cheese

DATE: Jan. 21, 2019

Current Season:

☐ **SPRING**
   the season of detox, renewal,
   lightening

☐ **SUMMER**
   the season of sun defense,
   hydration, activity

☐ **AUTUMN**
   the season of healing, balancing,
   grounding

☒ **WINTER**
   the season of nourishment, rest,
   preparation

Today's positive affirmation:
I am

in control of my life.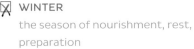

Today I am grateful for:

My career

Today's health and beauty goals:

wash face

Beauty Nutrition
Essentials I Enjoyed Today:

☐ Warm lemon water
☐ One or more servings of greens
☒ Seasonal fruit and veggies
☐ Protein and/or healthy fat
   at each meal
☐ Probiotics and/or fermented food
☒ Complete, mindful chewing at
   snack and mealtimes
☐ Fresh herbs and spices
☒ Regular meal intervals
☐ Frequent hydration
   (including ____ glasses of water)
☐ Supplements, if applicable
☐ Other:

Self-Care Essentials
I Enjoyed Today:

☒ Meditation and/or quiet time
☐ Deep breathing
☒ Physical activity
☒ Connection with friends
   or family
☐ De-stressing activity
☒ Self-love
☐ Beauty sleep (____ hours)
☐ Other:

DAILY FOOD DIARY

Breakfast
What I ate: 1 hard boiled egg
a few pieces of
sausage

Time: 8 wam Setting: home

How I felt after eating:
still hungry

Lunch Brown Rice
What I ate: Sausage
Shakshuka Sauce
Israeli salad.

Time: 11:30 Setting: work

How I felt after eating:
gassy
cramps
tired

Dinner vege barley soup
What I ate: Mushrooms
brown rice broccoli
salmon cauliflower

Time: __:__ Setting:

How I felt after eating:
• mostly full
• I think it needed more
flavor, but still good

Other
Today's snacks: half small kutka
2 coffees popcorn
M&Ms mandarin
cheese 70% Lindt ball

Favorite beauty foods I ate today:
Mushrooms Egg
Salmon
Brocc
Cauliflower

When did you look and feel your best today?
morning

Takeaways from today:
- feeling bloated - less meat
- gassy - less cheese

69

DATE: Jan 22, 2019

Current Season:

☐ **SPRING**
the season of detox, renewal, lightening

☐ **SUMMER**
the season of sun defense, hydration, activity

☐ **AUTUMN**
the season of healing, balancing, grounding

☒ **WINTER**
the season of nourishment, rest, preparation

Today's positive affirmation:

I am calm and filled with joy

Today I am grateful for:

my priviteded life to be able to have food in my fridge

Today's health and beauty goals:

Take out garbage
Take iron pill

Beauty Nutrition Essentials I Enjoyed Today:

☐ Warm lemon water
☒ One or more servings of greens
☒ Seasonal fruit and veggies
☒ Protein and/or healthy fat at each meal
☐ Probiotics and/or fermented food
☒ Complete, mindful chewing at snack and mealtimes
☐ Fresh herbs and spices
☒ Regular meal intervals
☒ Frequent hydration (including ____ glasses of water)
☒ Supplements, if applicable
☐ Other:

Self-Care Essentials I Enjoyed Today:

☒ Meditation and/or quiet time
☒ Deep breathing
☒ Physical activity
☒ Connection with friends or family
☒ De-stressing activity
☐ Self-love
☐ Beauty sleep (____ hours)
☐ Other:

DAILY FOOD DIARY

Breakfast
What I ate: Sausage
hard boiled egg
half avocado

Time 7:30 am   Setting: home @ table

How I felt after eating:
nourished
gassy

Lunch
What I ate: salmon
rice
broc. cauli

Time 12:00   Setting: work

How I felt after eating:
full
energized

Dinner
What I ate: Salmon
brown rice
brocc
cauli

Time 6:00   Setting: home

How I felt after eating:
energized
but still hungry

Other
Today's snacks: Banana
carrots
hummus
½ pita

Favorite beauty foods I ate today:

carrots   cauli
salmon   brocc
egg
avo

When did you look and feel your best today?
In the morning
when I went to gym

Takeaways from today:
feeling bloated + huge today

DATE: **Saturday, Jan 26**

Current Season:

☐ SPRING
the season of detox, renewal, lightening

☐ SUMMER
the season of sun defense, hydration, activity

☐ AUTUMN
the season of healing, balancing, grounding

☒ WINTER
the season of nourishment, rest, preparation

Today's positive affirmation:
I am *a strong + beautiful woman*

Today I am grateful for:
my mother + father

Today's health and beauty goals:
enjoy my life

Beauty Nutrition
Essentials I Enjoyed Today:

☐ Warm lemon water
☐ One or more servings of greens
☐ Seasonal fruit and veggies
☒ Protein and/or healthy fat
at each meal
☐ Probiotics and/or fermented food
☐ Complete, mindful chewing at
snack and mealtimes
☐ Fresh herbs and spices
☐ Regular meal intervals
☐ Frequent hydration
(including ____ glasses of water)
☐ Supplements, if applicable
☐ Other:

Self-Care Essentials
I Enjoyed Today:

☐ Meditation and/or quiet time
☐ Deep breathing
☐ Physical activity
☐ Connection with friends
or family
☐ De-stressing activity
☐ Self-love
☐ Beauty sleep (____ hours)
☐ Other:

my cycle: PMS

DAILY FOOD DIARY

Breakfast
What I ate: multi grain toast, avocado, 2 eggs, feta

Time 10:30 | Setting: home

How I felt after eating:
- satisfied
- good
- happy

Lunch
What I ate:

Time __:__ | Setting:

How I felt after eating:

Dinner
What I ate:

Time __:__ | Setting:

How I felt after eating:

Other
Today's snacks:

Favorite beauty foods I ate today:

_____ _____

_____ _____

_____ _____

_____ _____

When did you look and feel your best today?

_____

Takeaways from today:

DATE: Feb. 3

Current Season:

☐ **SPRING**
the season of detox, renewal, lightening

☐ **SUMMER**
the season of sun defense, hydration, activity

☐ **AUTUMN**
the season of healing, balancing, grounding

☒ **WINTER**
the season of nourishment, rest, preparation

Today's positive affirmation:
I am

Today I am grateful for:

Today's health and beauty goals:

Beauty Nutrition
Essentials I Enjoyed Today:

☐ Warm lemon water
☐ One or more servings of greens
☒ Seasonal fruit and veggies
☒ Protein and/or healthy fat at each meal
☐ Probiotics and/or fermented food
☐ Complete, mindful chewing at snack and mealtimes
☐ Fresh herbs and spices
☐ Regular meal intervals
☐ Frequent hydration (including ____ glasses of water)
☐ Supplements, if applicable
☐ Other:

Self-Care Essentials
I Enjoyed Today:

☐ Meditation and/or quiet time
☐ Deep breathing
☐ Physical activity
☒ Connection with friends or family
☒ De-stressing activity
☐ Self-love
☐ Beauty sleep (____ hours)
☐ Other:

DAILY FOOD DIARY

Breakfast

What I ate:

Mushroom, chorizo hasb from earls

Time __:__   Setting:

How I felt after eating:

very full

Lunch

What I ate:

- ceasar
- coffee

Time __:__   Setting:

How I felt after eating:

Dinner

What I ate:

Time __:__   Setting:

How I felt after eating:

Other

Today's snacks:

Favorite beauty foods I ate today:

_____ _____

_____ _____

_____ _____

_____ _____

When did you look and feel your best today?

_____

Takeaways from today:

DATE:

Current Season:

☐ **SPRING**
the season of detox, renewal, lightening

☐ **SUMMER**
the season of sun defense, hydration, activity

☐ **AUTUMN**
the season of healing, balancing, grounding

☐ **WINTER**
the season of nourishment, rest, preparation

Today's positive affirmation:
I am

Today I am grateful for:

Today's health and beauty goals:

Beauty Nutrition Essentials I Enjoyed Today:

☐ Warm lemon water
☐ One or more servings of greens
☐ Seasonal fruit and veggies
☐ Protein and/or healthy fat at each meal
☐ Probiotics and/or fermented food
☐ Complete, mindful chewing at snack and mealtimes
☐ Fresh herbs and spices
☐ Regular meal intervals
☐ Frequent hydration (including _____ glasses of water)
☐ Supplements, if applicable
☐ Other:

Self-Care Essentials I Enjoyed Today:

☐ Meditation and/or quiet time
☐ Deep breathing
☐ Physical activity
☐ Connection with friends or family
☐ De-stressing activity
☐ Self-love
☐ Beauty sleep (_____ hours)
☐ Other:

DAILY FOOD DIARY

Breakfast
What I ate:

Time __:__ | Setting:

How I felt after eating:

Lunch
What I ate:

Time __:__ | Setting:

How I felt after eating:

Dinner
What I ate:

Time __:__ | Setting:

How I felt after eating:

Other
Today's snacks:

Favorite beauty foods I ate today:

_____ _____

_____ _____

_____ _____

_____ _____

When did you look and feel your best today?

_____

Takeaways from today:

DATE:

Current Season:

☐ **SPRING**
the season of detox, renewal, lightening

☐ **SUMMER**
the season of sun defense, hydration, activity

☐ **AUTUMN**
the season of healing, balancing, grounding

☐ **WINTER**
the season of nourishment, rest, preparation

Today's positive affirmation:
I am

Today I am grateful for:

Today's health and beauty goals:

Beauty Nutrition Essentials I Enjoyed Today:

☐ Warm lemon water
☐ One or more servings of greens
☐ Seasonal fruit and veggies
☐ Protein and/or healthy fat at each meal
☐ Probiotics and/or fermented food
☐ Complete, mindful chewing at snack and mealtimes
☐ Fresh herbs and spices
☐ Regular meal intervals
☐ Frequent hydration (including ____ glasses of water)
☐ Supplements, if applicable
☐ Other:

Self-Care Essentials I Enjoyed Today:

☐ Meditation and/or quiet time
☐ Deep breathing
☐ Physical activity
☐ Connection with friends or family
☐ De-stressing activity
☐ Self-love
☐ Beauty sleep (____ hours)
☐ Other:

DAILY FOOD DIARY

Breakfast
What I ate:

Time __:__ | Setting:

How I felt after eating:

Lunch
What I ate:

Time __:__ | Setting:

How I felt after eating:

Dinner
What I ate:

Time __:__ | Setting:

How I felt after eating:

Other
Today's snacks:

Favorite beauty foods I ate today:

_____ _____

_____ _____

_____ _____

_____ _____

When did you look and feel your best today?

_____

Takeaways from today:

DATE:

Current Season:

☐ **SPRING**
the season of detox, renewal, lightening

☐ **SUMMER**
the season of sun defense, hydration, activity

☐ **AUTUMN**
the season of healing, balancing, grounding

☐ **WINTER**
the season of nourishment, rest, preparation

Today's positive affirmation:
I am

Today I am grateful for:

Today's health and beauty goals:

Beauty Nutrition Essentials I Enjoyed Today:

☐ Warm lemon water
☐ One or more servings of greens
☐ Seasonal fruit and veggies
☐ Protein and/or healthy fat at each meal
☐ Probiotics and/or fermented food
☐ Complete, mindful chewing at snack and mealtimes
☐ Fresh herbs and spices
☐ Regular meal intervals
☐ Frequent hydration (including ____ glasses of water)
☐ Supplements, if applicable
☐ Other:

Self-Care Essentials I Enjoyed Today:

☐ Meditation and/or quiet time
☐ Deep breathing
☐ Physical activity
☐ Connection with friends or family
☐ De-stressing activity
☐ Self-love
☐ Beauty sleep (____ hours)
☐ Other:

DAILY FOOD DIARY

Breakfast
What I ate:

Time __:__   Setting:

How I felt after eating:

Lunch
What I ate:

Time __:__   Setting:

How I felt after eating:

Dinner
What I ate:

Time __:__   Setting:

How I felt after eating:

Other
Today's snacks:

Favorite beauty foods I ate today:

_____   _____

_____   _____

_____   _____

_____   _____

When did you look and feel your best today?

_____

Takeaways from today:

DATE:

Current Season:

☐ **SPRING**
   the season of detox, renewal, lightening

☐ **SUMMER**
   the season of sun defense, hydration, activity

☐ **AUTUMN**
   the season of healing, balancing, grounding

☐ **WINTER**
   the season of nourishment, rest, preparation

Today's positive affirmation:

I am

Today I am grateful for:

Today's health and beauty goals:

Beauty Nutrition Essentials I Enjoyed Today:

☐ Warm lemon water
☐ One or more servings of greens
☐ Seasonal fruit and veggies
☐ Protein and/or healthy fat at each meal
☐ Probiotics and/or fermented food
☐ Complete, mindful chewing at snack and mealtimes
☐ Fresh herbs and spices
☐ Regular meal intervals
☐ Frequent hydration (including ____ glasses of water)
☐ Supplements, if applicable
☐ Other:

Self-Care Essentials I Enjoyed Today:

☐ Meditation and/or quiet time
☐ Deep breathing
☐ Physical activity
☐ Connection with friends or family
☐ De-stressing activity
☐ Self-love
☐ Beauty sleep (____ hours)
☐ Other:

DAILY FOOD DIARY

Breakfast
What I ate:

Time __:__ | Setting:

How I felt after eating:

Lunch
What I ate:

Time __:__ | Setting:

How I felt after eating:

Dinner
What I ate:

Time __:__ | Setting:

How I felt after eating:

Other
Today's snacks:

Favorite beauty foods I ate today:

_____ _____

_____ _____

_____ _____

_____ _____

When did you look and feel your best today?

_____

Takeaways from today:

DATE:

Current Season:

- [ ] **SPRING**
  the season of detox, renewal, lightening

- [ ] **SUMMER**
  the season of sun defense, hydration, activity

- [ ] **AUTUMN**
  the season of healing, balancing, grounding

- [ ] **WINTER**
  the season of nourishment, rest, preparation

Today's positive affirmation:
I am

Today I am grateful for:

Today's health and beauty goals:

Beauty Nutrition Essentials I Enjoyed Today:

- [ ] Warm lemon water
- [ ] One or more servings of greens
- [ ] Seasonal fruit and veggies
- [ ] Protein and/or healthy fat at each meal
- [ ] Probiotics and/or fermented food
- [ ] Complete, mindful chewing at snack and mealtimes
- [ ] Fresh herbs and spices
- [ ] Regular meal intervals
- [ ] Frequent hydration (including ____ glasses of water)
- [ ] Supplements, if applicable
- [ ] Other:

Self-Care Essentials I Enjoyed Today:

- [ ] Meditation and/or quiet time
- [ ] Deep breathing
- [ ] Physical activity
- [ ] Connection with friends or family
- [ ] De-stressing activity
- [ ] Self-love
- [ ] Beauty sleep (____ hours)
- [ ] Other:

DAILY FOOD DIARY

Breakfast
What I ate:

Time __:__ | Setting:

How I felt after eating:

Lunch
What I ate:

Time __:__ | Setting:

How I felt after eating:

Dinner
What I ate:

Time __:__ | Setting:

How I felt after eating:

Other
Today's snacks:

Favorite beauty foods I ate today:

_____ _____

_____ _____

_____ _____

_____ _____

When did you look and feel your best today?

_____

Takeaways from today:

A MOMENT TO CHECK IN

If you've reached this page, you've filled in ten journal entries. Take a moment to look back on what you've recorded and assess how your choices are impacting the way you look and feel. These questions will help you hone in on the foods and habits that are proving themselves to be most beneficial to your health and beauty, and point out adjustments that you may wish to make as you continue.

Describe the current state of your:

Skin	
Hair	
Nails	
Energy	
Weight	
Mood	
Resilience to Stress	

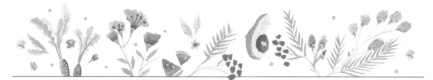

As you reflect on the previous journal entries, identify the following:

What new healthy habits did you cultivate during this period of journaling? What results did you see from these healthy habits?

Were there any new habits that didn't work well for you or didn't fit well into your lifestyle?

What challenges—including foods, thoughts, or habits—held you back from looking and feeling your best?

As you continue to build your new beautifying lifestyle, consider the following:

What are some new or developing beauty and health goals that you intend to focus on?

What are some challenges you foresee in the period ahead that might prevent you from meeting these goals?

Record words of encouragement or advice from yourself or others to inspire you along the way.

DATE:

Current Season:

☐ **SPRING**
   the season of detox, renewal, lightening

☐ **SUMMER**
   the season of sun defense, hydration, activity

☐ **AUTUMN**
   the season of healing, balancing, grounding

☐ **WINTER**
   the season of nourishment, rest, preparation

Today's positive affirmation:

I am

Today I am grateful for:

Today's health and beauty goals:

Beauty Nutrition Essentials I Enjoyed Today:

☐ Warm lemon water
☐ One or more servings of greens
☐ Seasonal fruit and veggies
☐ Protein and/or healthy fat at each meal
☐ Probiotics and/or fermented food
☐ Complete, mindful chewing at snack and mealtimes
☐ Fresh herbs and spices
☐ Regular meal intervals
☐ Frequent hydration (including ____ glasses of water)
☐ Supplements, if applicable
☐ Other:

Self-Care Essentials I Enjoyed Today:

☐ Meditation and/or quiet time
☐ Deep breathing
☐ Physical activity
☐ Connection with friends or family
☐ De-stressing activity
☐ Self-love
☐ Beauty sleep (____ hours)
☐ Other:

DAILY FOOD DIARY

Breakfast
What I ate:

Time __:__ | Setting:

How I felt after eating:

Lunch
What I ate:

Time __:__ | Setting:

How I felt after eating:

Dinner
What I ate:

Time __:__ | Setting:

How I felt after eating:

Other
Today's snacks:

Favorite beauty foods I ate today:

_____ _____

_____ _____

_____ _____

_____ _____

When did you look and feel your best today?

Takeaways from today:

DATE:

Current Season:

☐ **SPRING**
the season of detox, renewal, lightening

☐ **SUMMER**
the season of sun defense, hydration, activity

☐ **AUTUMN**
the season of healing, balancing, grounding

☐ **WINTER**
the season of nourishment, rest, preparation

Today's positive affirmation:
I am

Today I am grateful for:

Today's health and beauty goals:

Beauty Nutrition Essentials I Enjoyed Today:

☐ Warm lemon water
☐ One or more servings of greens
☐ Seasonal fruit and veggies
☐ Protein and/or healthy fat at each meal
☐ Probiotics and/or fermented food
☐ Complete, mindful chewing at snack and mealtimes
☐ Fresh herbs and spices
☐ Regular meal intervals
☐ Frequent hydration (including ____ glasses of water)
☐ Supplements, if applicable
☐ Other:

Self-Care Essentials I Enjoyed Today:

☐ Meditation and/or quiet time
☐ Deep breathing
☐ Physical activity
☐ Connection with friends or family
☐ De-stressing activity
☐ Self-love
☐ Beauty sleep (____ hours)
☐ Other:

DAILY FOOD DIARY

Breakfast
What I ate:

Time __:__   Setting:

How I felt after eating:

Lunch
What I ate:

Time __:__   Setting:

How I felt after eating:

Dinner
What I ate:

Time __:__   Setting:

How I felt after eating:

Other
Today's snacks:

Favorite beauty foods I ate today:

_____ _____

_____ _____

_____ _____

_____ _____

When did you look and feel your best today?

_____

Takeaways from today:

DATE:

Current Season:

☐ **SPRING**
the season of detox, renewal, lightening

☐ **SUMMER**
the season of sun defense, hydration, activity

☐ **AUTUMN**
the season of healing, balancing, grounding

☐ **WINTER**
the season of nourishment, rest, preparation

Today's positive affirmation:
I am

Today I am grateful for:

Today's health and beauty goals:

Beauty Nutrition Essentials I Enjoyed Today:

☐ Warm lemon water
☐ One or more servings of greens
☐ Seasonal fruit and veggies
☐ Protein and/or healthy fat at each meal
☐ Probiotics and/or fermented food
☐ Complete, mindful chewing at snack and mealtimes
☐ Fresh herbs and spices
☐ Regular meal intervals
☐ Frequent hydration (including ____ glasses of water)
☐ Supplements, if applicable
☐ Other:

Self-Care Essentials I Enjoyed Today:

☐ Meditation and/or quiet time
☐ Deep breathing
☐ Physical activity
☐ Connection with friends or family
☐ De-stressing activity
☐ Self-love
☐ Beauty sleep (____ hours)
☐ Other:

DAILY FOOD DIARY

Breakfast
What I ate:

Time __:__ | Setting:

How I felt after eating:

Lunch
What I ate:

Time __:__ | Setting:

How I felt after eating:

Dinner
What I ate:

Time __:__ | Setting:

How I felt after eating:

Other
Today's snacks:

Favorite beauty foods I ate today:

_____ _____

_____ _____

_____ _____

_____ _____

When did you look and feel your best today?

_____

Takeaways from today:

DATE:

Current Season:

- ☐ **SPRING**
  the season of detox, renewal, lightening

- ☐ **SUMMER**
  the season of sun defense, hydration, activity

- ☐ **AUTUMN**
  the season of healing, balancing, grounding

- ☐ **WINTER**
  the season of nourishment, rest, preparation

Today's positive affirmation:

I am

Today I am grateful for:

Today's health and beauty goals:

Beauty Nutrition Essentials I Enjoyed Today:

- ☐ Warm lemon water
- ☐ One or more servings of greens
- ☐ Seasonal fruit and veggies
- ☐ Protein and/or healthy fat at each meal
- ☐ Probiotics and/or fermented food
- ☐ Complete, mindful chewing at snack and mealtimes
- ☐ Fresh herbs and spices
- ☐ Regular meal intervals
- ☐ Frequent hydration (including ____ glasses of water)
- ☐ Supplements, if applicable
- ☐ Other:

Self-Care Essentials I Enjoyed Today:

- ☐ Meditation and/or quiet time
- ☐ Deep breathing
- ☐ Physical activity
- ☐ Connection with friends or family
- ☐ De-stressing activity
- ☐ Self-love
- ☐ Beauty sleep (____ hours)
- ☐ Other:

DAILY FOOD DIARY

Breakfast
What I ate:

Time __:__ | Setting:

How I felt after eating:

Lunch
What I ate:

Time __:__ | Setting:

How I felt after eating:

Dinner
What I ate:

Time __:__ | Setting:

How I felt after eating:

Other
Today's snacks:

Favorite beauty foods I ate today:

_____ _____

_____ _____

_____ _____

_____ _____

When did you look and feel your best today?

_____

Takeaways from today:

DATE:

Current Season:

☐ **SPRING**
the season of detox, renewal, lightening

☐ **SUMMER**
the season of sun defense, hydration, activity

☐ **AUTUMN**
the season of healing, balancing, grounding

☐ **WINTER**
the season of nourishment, rest, preparation

Today's positive affirmation:
I am

Today I am grateful for:

Today's health and beauty goals:

Beauty Nutrition Essentials I Enjoyed Today:

☐ Warm lemon water
☐ One or more servings of greens
☐ Seasonal fruit and veggies
☐ Protein and/or healthy fat at each meal
☐ Probiotics and/or fermented food
☐ Complete, mindful chewing at snack and mealtimes
☐ Fresh herbs and spices
☐ Regular meal intervals
☐ Frequent hydration (including ____ glasses of water)
☐ Supplements, if applicable
☐ Other:

Self-Care Essentials I Enjoyed Today:

☐ Meditation and/or quiet time
☐ Deep breathing
☐ Physical activity
☐ Connection with friends or family
☐ De-stressing activity
☐ Self-love
☐ Beauty sleep (____ hours)
☐ Other:

DAILY FOOD DIARY

Breakfast
What I ate:

Time __:__ | Setting:

How I felt after eating:

Lunch
What I ate:

Time __:__ | Setting:

How I felt after eating:

Dinner
What I ate:

Time __:__ | Setting:

How I felt after eating:

Other
Today's snacks:

Favorite beauty foods I ate today:

_____ _____

_____ _____

_____ _____

_____ _____

When did you look and feel your best today?

_____

Takeaways from today:

DATE:

Current Season:

☐ **SPRING**
the season of detox, renewal, lightening

☐ **SUMMER**
the season of sun defense, hydration, activity

☐ **AUTUMN**
the season of healing, balancing, grounding

☐ **WINTER**
the season of nourishment, rest, preparation

Today's positive affirmation:
I am

Today I am grateful for:

Today's health and beauty goals:

Beauty Nutrition
Essentials I Enjoyed Today:

☐ Warm lemon water
☐ One or more servings of greens
☐ Seasonal fruit and veggies
☐ Protein and/or healthy fat
at each meal
☐ Probiotics and/or fermented food
☐ Complete, mindful chewing at
snack and mealtimes
☐ Fresh herbs and spices
☐ Regular meal intervals
☐ Frequent hydration
(including ____ glasses of water)
☐ Supplements, if applicable
☐ Other:

Self-Care Essentials
I Enjoyed Today:

☐ Meditation and/or quiet time
☐ Deep breathing
☐ Physical activity
☐ Connection with friends
or family
☐ De-stressing activity
☐ Self-love
☐ Beauty sleep (____ hours)
☐ Other:

DAILY FOOD DIARY

Breakfast
What I ate:

Time __:__ | Setting:

How I felt after eating:

Lunch
What I ate:

Time __:__ | Setting:

How I felt after eating:

Dinner
What I ate:

Time __:__ | Setting:

How I felt after eating:

Other
Today's snacks:

Favorite beauty foods I ate today:

_____ _____

_____ _____

_____ _____

_____ _____

When did you look and feel your best today?

_____

Takeaways from today:

DATE:

Current Season:

☐ **SPRING**
the season of detox, renewal, lightening

☐ **SUMMER**
the season of sun defense, hydration, activity

☐ **AUTUMN**
the season of healing, balancing, grounding

☐ **WINTER**
the season of nourishment, rest, preparation

Today's positive affirmation:
I am

Today I am grateful for:

Today's health and beauty goals:

Beauty Nutrition
Essentials I Enjoyed Today:

☐ Warm lemon water
☐ One or more servings of greens
☐ Seasonal fruit and veggies
☐ Protein and/or healthy fat
   at each meal
☐ Probiotics and/or fermented food
☐ Complete, mindful chewing at
   snack and mealtimes
☐ Fresh herbs and spices
☐ Regular meal intervals
☐ Frequent hydration
   (including ____ glasses of water)
☐ Supplements, if applicable
☐ Other:

Self-Care Essentials
I Enjoyed Today:

☐ Meditation and/or quiet time
☐ Deep breathing
☐ Physical activity
☐ Connection with friends
   or family
☐ De-stressing activity
☐ Self-love
☐ Beauty sleep (____ hours)
☐ Other:

DAILY FOOD DIARY

Breakfast
What I ate:

Time __:__   Setting:

How I felt after eating:

Lunch
What I ate:

Time __:__   Setting:

How I felt after eating:

Dinner
What I ate:

Time __:__   Setting:

How I felt after eating:

Other
Today's snacks:

Favorite beauty foods I ate today:

_____   _____

_____   _____

_____   _____

_____   _____

When did you look and feel your best today?

_____

Takeaways from today:

DATE:

Current Season:

- [ ] **SPRING**
  the season of detox, renewal, lightening
- [ ] **SUMMER**
  the season of sun defense, hydration, activity
- [ ] **AUTUMN**
  the season of healing, balancing, grounding
- [ ] **WINTER**
  the season of nourishment, rest, preparation

Today's positive affirmation:

I am

Today I am grateful for:

Today's health and beauty goals:

Beauty Nutrition Essentials I Enjoyed Today:

- [ ] Warm lemon water
- [ ] One or more servings of greens
- [ ] Seasonal fruit and veggies
- [ ] Protein and/or healthy fat at each meal
- [ ] Probiotics and/or fermented food
- [ ] Complete, mindful chewing at snack and mealtimes
- [ ] Fresh herbs and spices
- [ ] Regular meal intervals
- [ ] Frequent hydration (including ____ glasses of water)
- [ ] Supplements, if applicable
- [ ] Other:

Self-Care Essentials I Enjoyed Today:

- [ ] Meditation and/or quiet time
- [ ] Deep breathing
- [ ] Physical activity
- [ ] Connection with friends or family
- [ ] De-stressing activity
- [ ] Self-love
- [ ] Beauty sleep (____ hours)
- [ ] Other:

DAILY FOOD DIARY

Breakfast
What I ate:

Time __:__ | Setting:

How I felt after eating:

Lunch
What I ate:

Time __:__ | Setting:

How I felt after eating:

Dinner
What I ate:

Time __:__ | Setting:

How I felt after eating:

Other
Today's snacks:

Favorite beauty foods I ate today:

_____ _____

_____ _____

_____ _____

_____ _____

When did you look and feel your best today?

_____

Takeaways from today:

DATE:

Current Season:

- ☐ **SPRING**
  the season of detox, renewal, lightening
- ☐ **SUMMER**
  the season of sun defense, hydration, activity
- ☐ **AUTUMN**
  the season of healing, balancing, grounding
- ☐ **WINTER**
  the season of nourishment, rest, preparation

Today's positive affirmation:
I am

Today I am grateful for:

Today's health and beauty goals:

Beauty Nutrition
Essentials I Enjoyed Today:

- ☐ Warm lemon water
- ☐ One or more servings of greens
- ☐ Seasonal fruit and veggies
- ☐ Protein and/or healthy fat at each meal
- ☐ Probiotics and/or fermented food
- ☐ Complete, mindful chewing at snack and mealtimes
- ☐ Fresh herbs and spices
- ☐ Regular meal intervals
- ☐ Frequent hydration (including ____ glasses of water)
- ☐ Supplements, if applicable
- ☐ Other:

Self-Care Essentials
I Enjoyed Today:

- ☐ Meditation and/or quiet time
- ☐ Deep breathing
- ☐ Physical activity
- ☐ Connection with friends or family
- ☐ De-stressing activity
- ☐ Self-love
- ☐ Beauty sleep (____ hours)
- ☐ Other:

DAILY FOOD DIARY

Breakfast
What I ate:

Time __:__ | Setting:

How I felt after eating:

Lunch
What I ate:

Time __:__ | Setting:

How I felt after eating:

Dinner
What I ate:

Time __:__ | Setting:

How I felt after eating:

Other
Today's snacks:

Favorite beauty foods I ate today:

_____ _____

_____ _____

_____ _____

When did you look and feel your best today?

_____

Takeaways from today:

DATE:

Current Season:

☐ **SPRING**
the season of detox, renewal, lightening

☐ **SUMMER**
the season of sun defense, hydration, activity

☐ **AUTUMN**
the season of healing, balancing, grounding

☐ **WINTER**
the season of nourishment, rest, preparation

Today's positive affirmation:
I am

Today I am grateful for:

Today's health and beauty goals:

Beauty Nutrition Essentials I Enjoyed Today:

☐ Warm lemon water
☐ One or more servings of greens
☐ Seasonal fruit and veggies
☐ Protein and/or healthy fat at each meal
☐ Probiotics and/or fermented food
☐ Complete, mindful chewing at snack and mealtimes
☐ Fresh herbs and spices
☐ Regular meal intervals
☐ Frequent hydration (including ___ glasses of water)
☐ Supplements, if applicable
☐ Other:

Self-Care Essentials I Enjoyed Today:

☐ Meditation and/or quiet time
☐ Deep breathing
☐ Physical activity
☐ Connection with friends or family
☐ De-stressing activity
☐ Self-love
☐ Beauty sleep (___ hours)
☐ Other:

DAILY FOOD DIARY

Breakfast
What I ate:

Time __:__ | Setting:

How I felt after eating:

Lunch
What I ate:

Time __:__ | Setting:

How I felt after eating:

Dinner
What I ate:

Time __:__ | Setting:

How I felt after eating:

Other
Today's snacks:

Favorite beauty foods I ate today:

_____ _____

_____ _____

_____ _____

_____ _____

When did you look and feel your best today?

_____

Takeaways from today:

➤ A MOMENT TO CHECK IN ⭠

If you've reached this page, you've filled in ten journal entries. Take a moment to look back on what you've recorded and assess how your choices are impacting the way you look and feel. These questions will help you hone in on the foods and habits that are proving themselves to be most beneficial to your health and beauty, and point out adjustments that you may wish to make as you continue.

Describe the current state of your:

Skin	
Hair	
Nails	
Energy	
Weight	
Mood	
Resilience to Stress	

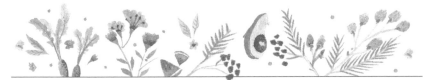

As you reflect on the previous journal entries, identify the following:

What new healthy habits did you cultivate during this period of journaling? What results did you see from these healthy habits?

Were there any new habits that didn't work well for you or didn't fit well into your lifestyle?

What challenges—including foods, thoughts, or habits—held you back from looking and feeling your best?

As you continue to build your new beautifying lifestyle, consider the following:

What are some new or developing beauty and health goals that you intend to focus on?

What are some challenges you foresee in the period ahead that might prevent you from meeting these goals?

Record words of encouragement or advice from yourself or others to inspire you along the way.

DATE:

Current Season:

☐ **SPRING**
the season of detox, renewal, lightening

☐ **SUMMER**
the season of sun defense, hydration, activity

☐ **AUTUMN**
the season of healing, balancing, grounding

☐ **WINTER**
the season of nourishment, rest, preparation

Today's positive affirmation:
I am

Today I am grateful for:

Today's health and beauty goals:

Beauty Nutrition Essentials I Enjoyed Today:

☐ Warm lemon water
☐ One or more servings of greens
☐ Seasonal fruit and veggies
☐ Protein and/or healthy fat at each meal
☐ Probiotics and/or fermented food
☐ Complete, mindful chewing at snack and mealtimes
☐ Fresh herbs and spices
☐ Regular meal intervals
☐ Frequent hydration (including ____ glasses of water)
☐ Supplements, if applicable
☐ Other:

Self-Care Essentials I Enjoyed Today:

☐ Meditation and/or quiet time
☐ Deep breathing
☐ Physical activity
☐ Connection with friends or family
☐ De-stressing activity
☐ Self-love
☐ Beauty sleep (____ hours)
☐ Other:

DAILY FOOD DIARY

Breakfast
What I ate:

Time __:__   Setting:

How I felt after eating:

Lunch
What I ate:

Time __:__   Setting:

How I felt after eating:

Dinner
What I ate:

Time __:__   Setting:

How I felt after eating:

Other
Today's snacks:

Favorite beauty foods I ate today:

_____ _____

_____ _____

_____ _____

_____ _____

When did you look and feel your best today?

_____

Takeaways from today:

DATE:

Current Season:

- ☐ **SPRING**
  the season of detox, renewal, lightening
- ☐ **SUMMER**
  the season of sun defense, hydration, activity
- ☐ **AUTUMN**
  the season of healing, balancing, grounding
- ☐ **WINTER**
  the season of nourishment, rest, preparation

Today's positive affirmation:

I am

Today I am grateful for:

Today's health and beauty goals:

Beauty Nutrition Essentials I Enjoyed Today:

- ☐ Warm lemon water
- ☐ One or more servings of greens
- ☐ Seasonal fruit and veggies
- ☐ Protein and/or healthy fat at each meal
- ☐ Probiotics and/or fermented food
- ☐ Complete, mindful chewing at snack and mealtimes
- ☐ Fresh herbs and spices
- ☐ Regular meal intervals
- ☐ Frequent hydration (including ____ glasses of water)
- ☐ Supplements, if applicable
- ☐ Other:

Self-Care Essentials I Enjoyed Today:

- ☐ Meditation and/or quiet time
- ☐ Deep breathing
- ☐ Physical activity
- ☐ Connection with friends or family
- ☐ De-stressing activity
- ☐ Self-love
- ☐ Beauty sleep (____ hours)
- ☐ Other:

DAILY FOOD DIARY

Breakfast
What I ate:

Time __:__ | Setting:

How I felt after eating:

Lunch
What I ate:

Time __:__ | Setting:

How I felt after eating:

Dinner
What I ate:

Time __:__ | Setting:

How I felt after eating:

Other
Today's snacks:

Favorite beauty foods I ate today:

_____ _____

_____ _____

_____ _____

_____ _____

When did you look and feel your best today?

Takeaways from today:

DATE:

Current Season:

☐ **SPRING**
   the season of detox, renewal, lightening

☐ **SUMMER**
   the season of sun defense, hydration, activity

☐ **AUTUMN**
   the season of healing, balancing, grounding

☐ **WINTER**
   the season of nourishment, rest, preparation

Today's positive affirmation:
I am

Today I am grateful for:

Today's health and beauty goals:

Beauty Nutrition Essentials I Enjoyed Today:

☐ Warm lemon water
☐ One or more servings of greens
☐ Seasonal fruit and veggies
☐ Protein and/or healthy fat at each meal
☐ Probiotics and/or fermented food
☐ Complete, mindful chewing at snack and mealtimes
☐ Fresh herbs and spices
☐ Regular meal intervals
☐ Frequent hydration (including ____ glasses of water)
☐ Supplements, if applicable
☐ Other:

Self-Care Essentials I Enjoyed Today:

☐ Meditation and/or quiet time
☐ Deep breathing
☐ Physical activity
☐ Connection with friends or family
☐ De-stressing activity
☐ Self-love
☐ Beauty sleep (____ hours)
☐ Other:

DAILY FOOD DIARY

Breakfast
What I ate:

Time __:__   Setting:

How I felt after eating:

Lunch
What I ate:

Time __:__   Setting:

How I felt after eating:

Dinner
What I ate:

Time __:__   Setting:

How I felt after eating:

Other
Today's snacks:

Favorite beauty foods I ate today:

_____   _____

_____   _____

_____   _____

_____   _____

When did you look and feel your best today?

_____

Takeaways from today:

DATE:

Current Season:

☐ **SPRING**
   the season of detox, renewal, lightening

☐ **SUMMER**
   the season of sun defense, hydration, activity

☐ **AUTUMN**
   the season of healing, balancing, grounding

☐ **WINTER**
   the season of nourishment, rest, preparation

Today's positive affirmation:
I am

Today I am grateful for:

Today's health and beauty goals:

Beauty Nutrition Essentials I Enjoyed Today:

☐ Warm lemon water
☐ One or more servings of greens
☐ Seasonal fruit and veggies
☐ Protein and/or healthy fat at each meal
☐ Probiotics and/or fermented food
☐ Complete, mindful chewing at snack and mealtimes
☐ Fresh herbs and spices
☐ Regular meal intervals
☐ Frequent hydration (including ____ glasses of water)
☐ Supplements, if applicable
☐ Other:

Self-Care Essentials I Enjoyed Today:

☐ Meditation and/or quiet time
☐ Deep breathing
☐ Physical activity
☐ Connection with friends or family
☐ De-stressing activity
☐ Self-love
☐ Beauty sleep (____ hours)
☐ Other:

DAILY FOOD DIARY

Breakfast
What I ate:

Time __:__ | Setting:

How I felt after eating:

Lunch
What I ate:

Time __:__ | Setting:

How I felt after eating:

Dinner
What I ate:

Time __:__ | Setting:

How I felt after eating:

Other
Today's snacks:

Favorite beauty foods I ate today:

_____ _____

_____ _____

_____ _____

_____ _____

When did you look and feel your best today?

_____

Takeaways from today:

DATE:

Current Season:

☐ **SPRING**
   the season of detox, renewal,
   lightening

☐ **SUMMER**
   the season of sun defense,
   hydration, activity

☐ **AUTUMN**
   the season of healing, balancing,
   grounding

☐ **WINTER**
   the season of nourishment, rest,
   preparation

Today's positive affirmation:
I am

Today I am grateful for:

Today's health and beauty goals:

Beauty Nutrition Essentials I Enjoyed Today:

☐ Warm lemon water
☐ One or more servings of greens
☐ Seasonal fruit and veggies
☐ Protein and/or healthy fat
   at each meal
☐ Probiotics and/or fermented food
☐ Complete, mindful chewing at
   snack and mealtimes
☐ Fresh herbs and spices
☐ Regular meal intervals
☐ Frequent hydration
   (including ____ glasses of water)
☐ Supplements, if applicable
☐ Other:

Self-Care Essentials I Enjoyed Today:

☐ Meditation and/or quiet time
☐ Deep breathing
☐ Physical activity
☐ Connection with friends
   or family
☐ De-stressing activity
☐ Self-love
☐ Beauty sleep (____ hours)
☐ Other:

DAILY FOOD DIARY

Breakfast
What I ate:

Time __:__   Setting:

How I felt after eating:

Lunch
What I ate:

Time __:__   Setting:

How I felt after eating:

Dinner
What I ate:

Time __:__   Setting:

How I felt after eating:

Other
Today's snacks:

Favorite beauty foods I ate today:

_____   _____

_____   _____

_____   _____

_____   _____

When did you look and feel your best today?

_____

Takeaways from today:

DATE:

Current Season:

☐ **SPRING**
the season of detox, renewal, lightening

☐ **SUMMER**
the season of sun defense, hydration, activity

☐ **AUTUMN**
the season of healing, balancing, grounding

☐ **WINTER**
the season of nourishment, rest, preparation

Today's positive affirmation:
I am

Today I am grateful for:

Today's health and beauty goals:

Beauty Nutrition Essentials I Enjoyed Today:

☐ Warm lemon water
☐ One or more servings of greens
☐ Seasonal fruit and veggies
☐ Protein and/or healthy fat at each meal
☐ Probiotics and/or fermented food
☐ Complete, mindful chewing at snack and mealtimes
☐ Fresh herbs and spices
☐ Regular meal intervals
☐ Frequent hydration (including ____ glasses of water)
☐ Supplements, if applicable
☐ Other:

Self-Care Essentials I Enjoyed Today:

☐ Meditation and/or quiet time
☐ Deep breathing
☐ Physical activity
☐ Connection with friends or family
☐ De-stressing activity
☐ Self-love
☐ Beauty sleep (____ hours)
☐ Other:

DAILY FOOD DIARY

Breakfast
What I ate:

Time __:__ | Setting:

How I felt after eating:

Lunch
What I ate:

Time __:__ | Setting:

How I felt after eating:

Dinner
What I ate:

Time __:__ | Setting:

How I felt after eating:

Other
Today's snacks:

Favorite beauty foods I ate today:

_____ _____

_____ _____

_____ _____

_____ _____

When did you look and feel your best today?

_____

Takeaways from today:

DATE:

Current Season:

☐ **SPRING**
    the season of detox, renewal, lightening

☐ **SUMMER**
    the season of sun defense, hydration, activity

☐ **AUTUMN**
    the season of healing, balancing, grounding

☐ **WINTER**
    the season of nourishment, rest, preparation

Today's positive affirmation:

I am

Today I am grateful for:

Today's health and beauty goals:

**Beauty Nutrition
Essentials I Enjoyed Today:**

☐ Warm lemon water
☐ One or more servings of greens
☐ Seasonal fruit and veggies
☐ Protein and/or healthy fat
    at each meal
☐ Probiotics and/or fermented food
☐ Complete, mindful chewing at
    snack and mealtimes
☐ Fresh herbs and spices
☐ Regular meal intervals
☐ Frequent hydration
    (including _____ glasses of water)
☐ Supplements, if applicable
☐ Other:

**Self-Care Essentials
I Enjoyed Today:**

☐ Meditation and/or quiet time
☐ Deep breathing
☐ Physical activity
☐ Connection with friends
    or family
☐ De-stressing activity
☐ Self-love
☐ Beauty sleep (_____ hours)
☐ Other:

DAILY FOOD DIARY

Breakfast
What I ate.

Time __:__ | Setting:

How I felt after eating:

Lunch
What I ate:

Time __:__ | Setting:

How I felt after eating:

Dinner
What I ate:

Time __:__ | Setting:

How I felt after eating:

Other
Today's snacks:

Favorite beauty foods I ate today:

_____ _____

_____ _____

_____ _____

_____ _____

When did you look and feel your best today?

_____

Takeaways from today:

DATE:

Current Season:

- ☐ **SPRING**
  the season of detox, renewal, lightening
- ☐ **SUMMER**
  the season of sun defense, hydration, activity
- ☐ **AUTUMN**
  the season of healing, balancing, grounding
- ☐ **WINTER**
  the season of nourishment, rest, preparation

Today's positive affirmation:

I am

Today I am grateful for:

Today's health and beauty goals:

Beauty Nutrition Essentials I Enjoyed Today:

- ☐ Warm lemon water
- ☐ One or more servings of greens
- ☐ Seasonal fruit and veggies
- ☐ Protein and/or healthy fat at each meal
- ☐ Probiotics and/or fermented food
- ☐ Complete, mindful chewing at snack and mealtimes
- ☐ Fresh herbs and spices
- ☐ Regular meal intervals
- ☐ Frequent hydration (including ____ glasses of water)
- ☐ Supplements, if applicable
- ☐ Other:

Self-Care Essentials I Enjoyed Today:

- ☐ Meditation and/or quiet time
- ☐ Deep breathing
- ☐ Physical activity
- ☐ Connection with friends or family
- ☐ De-stressing activity
- ☐ Self-love
- ☐ Beauty sleep (____ hours)
- ☐ Other:

DAILY FOOD DIARY

Breakfast
What I ate:

Time __:__ | Setting:

How I felt after eating:

Lunch
What I ate:

Time __:__ | Setting:

How I felt after eating:

Dinner
What I ate:

Time __:__ | Setting:

How I felt after eating:

Other
Today's snacks:

Favorite beauty foods I ate today:

_____ _____

_____ _____

_____ _____

_____ _____

When did you look and feel your best today?

Takeaways from today:

DATE:

Current Season:

☐ **SPRING**
the season of detox, renewal, lightening

☐ **SUMMER**
the season of sun defense, hydration, activity

☐ **AUTUMN**
the season of healing, balancing, grounding

☐ **WINTER**
the season of nourishment, rest, preparation

Today's positive affirmation:
I am

Today I am grateful for:

Today's health and beauty goals:

Beauty Nutrition Essentials I Enjoyed Today:

☐ Warm lemon water
☐ One or more servings of greens
☐ Seasonal fruit and veggies
☐ Protein and/or healthy fat at each meal
☐ Probiotics and/or fermented food
☐ Complete, mindful chewing at snack and mealtimes
☐ Fresh herbs and spices
☐ Regular meal intervals
☐ Frequent hydration (including ____ glasses of water)
☐ Supplements, if applicable
☐ Other:

Self-Care Essentials I Enjoyed Today:

☐ Meditation and/or quiet time
☐ Deep breathing
☐ Physical activity
☐ Connection with friends or family
☐ De-stressing activity
☐ Self-love
☐ Beauty sleep (____ hours)
☐ Other:

DAILY FOOD DIARY

Breakfast
What I ate:

Time __:__ | Setting:

How I felt after eating:

Lunch
What I ate:

Time __:__ | Setting:

How I felt after eating:

Dinner
What I ate:

Time __:__ | Setting:

How I felt after eating:

Other
Today's snacks:

Favorite beauty foods I ate today:

_____ _____

_____ _____

_____ _____

_____ _____

When did you look and feel your best today?

Takeaways from today:

DATE:

Current Season:

☐ **SPRING**
the season of detox, renewal, lightening

☐ **SUMMER**
the season of sun defense, hydration, activity

☐ **AUTUMN**
the season of healing, balancing, grounding

☐ **WINTER**
the season of nourishment, rest, preparation

Today's positive affirmation:
I am

Today I am grateful for:

Today's health and beauty goals:

Beauty Nutrition
Essentials I Enjoyed Today:

☐ Warm lemon water
☐ One or more servings of greens
☐ Seasonal fruit and veggies
☐ Protein and/or healthy fat
   at each meal
☐ Probiotics and/or fermented food
☐ Complete, mindful chewing at
   snack and mealtimes
☐ Fresh herbs and spices
☐ Regular meal intervals
☐ Frequent hydration
   (including ___ glasses of water)
☐ Supplements, if applicable
☐ Other:

Self-Care Essentials
I Enjoyed Today:

☐ Meditation and/or quiet time
☐ Deep breathing
☐ Physical activity
☐ Connection with friends
   or family
☐ De-stressing activity
☐ Self-love
☐ Beauty sleep (___ hours)
☐ Other:

DAILY FOOD DIARY

Breakfast
What I ate:

Time __:__ | Setting:

How I felt after eating:

Lunch
What I ate:

Time __:__ | Setting:

How I felt after eating:

Dinner
What I ate:

Time __:__ | Setting:

How I felt after eating:

Other
Today's snacks:

Favorite beauty foods I ate today:

_____ _____

_____ _____

_____ _____

When did you look and feel your best today?

_____

Takeaways from today:

A MOMENT TO CHECK IN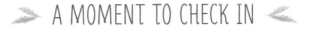

If you've reached this page, you've filled in ten journal entries. Take a moment to look back on what you've recorded and assess how your choices are impacting the way you look and feel. These questions will help you hone in on the foods and habits that are proving themselves to be most beneficial to your health and beauty, and point out adjustments that you may wish to make as you continue.

Describe the current state of your:

Skin	
Hair	
Nails	
Energy	
Weight	
Mood	
Resilience to Stress	

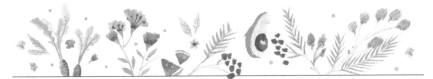

As you reflect on the previous journal entries, identify the following:

What new healthy habits did you cultivate during this period of journaling? What results did you see from these healthy habits?

Were there any new habits that didn't work well for you or didn't fit well into your lifestyle?

What challenges—including foods, thoughts, or habits—held you back from looking and feeling your best?

As you continue to build your new beautifying lifestyle, consider the following:

What are some new or developing beauty and health goals that you intend to focus on?

What are some challenges you foresee in the period ahead that might prevent you from meeting these goals?

Record words of encouragement or advice from yourself or others to inspire you along the way.

DATE:

Current Season:

☐ **SPRING**
the season of detox, renewal, lightening

☐ **SUMMER**
the season of sun defense, hydration, activity

☐ **AUTUMN**
the season of healing, balancing, grounding

☐ **WINTER**
the season of nourishment, rest, preparation

Today's positive affirmation:
I am

Today I am grateful for:

Today's health and beauty goals:

**Beauty Nutrition
Essentials I Enjoyed Today:**

☐ Warm lemon water
☐ One or more servings of greens
☐ Seasonal fruit and veggies
☐ Protein and/or healthy fat
at each meal
☐ Probiotics and/or fermented food
☐ Complete, mindful chewing at
snack and mealtimes
☐ Fresh herbs and spices
☐ Regular meal intervals
☐ Frequent hydration
(including ____ glasses of water)
☐ Supplements, if applicable
☐ Other:

**Self-Care Essentials
I Enjoyed Today:**

☐ Meditation and/or quiet time
☐ Deep breathing
☐ Physical activity
☐ Connection with friends
or family
☐ De-stressing activity
☐ Self-love
☐ Beauty sleep (____ hours)
☐ Other:

DAILY FOOD DIARY

Breakfast
What I ate:

Time __:__ | Setting:

How I felt after eating:

Lunch
What I ate:

Time __:__ | Setting:

How I felt after eating:

Dinner
What I ate:

Time __:__ | Setting:

How I felt after eating:

Other
Today's snacks:

Favorite beauty foods I ate today:

_____ _____

_____ _____

_____ _____

_____ _____

When did you look and feel your best today?

_____

Takeaways from today:

DATE:

Current Season:

☐ **SPRING**
the season of detox, renewal, lightening

☐ **SUMMER**
the season of sun defense, hydration, activity

☐ **AUTUMN**
the season of healing, balancing, grounding

☐ **WINTER**
the season of nourishment, rest, preparation

Today's positive affirmation:

I am

Today I am grateful for:

Today's health and beauty goals:

Beauty Nutrition
Essentials I Enjoyed Today:

☐ Warm lemon water
☐ One or more servings of greens
☐ Seasonal fruit and veggies
☐ Protein and/or healthy fat at each meal
☐ Probiotics and/or fermented food
☐ Complete, mindful chewing at snack and mealtimes
☐ Fresh herbs and spices
☐ Regular meal intervals
☐ Frequent hydration (including ____ glasses of water)
☐ Supplements, if applicable
☐ Other:

Self-Care Essentials
I Enjoyed Today:

☐ Meditation and/or quiet time
☐ Deep breathing
☐ Physical activity
☐ Connection with friends or family
☐ De-stressing activity
☐ Self-love
☐ Beauty sleep (____ hours)
☐ Other:

DAILY FOOD DIARY

Breakfast
What I ate:

Time __:__ | Setting:

How I felt after eating:

Lunch
What I ate:

Time __:__ | Setting:

How I felt after eating:

Dinner
What I ate:

Time __:__ | Setting:

How I felt after eating:

Other
Today's snacks:

Favorite beauty foods I ate today:

_____ _____

_____ _____

_____ _____

_____ _____

When did you look and feel your best today?

_____

Takeaways from today:

DATE:

Current Season:

☐ **SPRING**
the season of detox, renewal, lightening

☐ **SUMMER**
the season of sun defense, hydration, activity

☐ **AUTUMN**
the season of healing, balancing, grounding

☐ **WINTER**
the season of nourishment, rest, preparation

Today's positive affirmation:
I am

Today I am grateful for:

Today's health and beauty goals:

Beauty Nutrition Essentials I Enjoyed Today:

☐ Warm lemon water
☐ One or more servings of greens
☐ Seasonal fruit and veggies
☐ Protein and/or healthy fat at each meal
☐ Probiotics and/or fermented food
☐ Complete, mindful chewing at snack and mealtimes
☐ Fresh herbs and spices
☐ Regular meal intervals
☐ Frequent hydration (including ____ glasses of water)
☐ Supplements, if applicable
☐ Other:

Self-Care Essentials I Enjoyed Today:

☐ Meditation and/or quiet time
☐ Deep breathing
☐ Physical activity
☐ Connection with friends or family
☐ De-stressing activity
☐ Self-love
☐ Beauty sleep (____ hours)
☐ Other:

DAILY FOOD DIARY

Breakfast
What I ate:

Time __:__ | Setting:

How I felt after eating:

Lunch
What I ate:

Time __:__ | Setting:

How I felt after eating:

Dinner
What I ate:

Time __:__ | Setting:

How I felt after eating:

Other
Today's snacks:

Favorite beauty foods I ate today:

_____ _____

_____ _____

_____ _____

_____ _____

When did you look and feel your best today?

_____

Takeaways from today:

DATE:

Current Season:

☐ **SPRING**
the season of detox, renewal, lightening

☐ **SUMMER**
the season of sun defense, hydration, activity

☐ **AUTUMN**
the season of healing, balancing, grounding

☐ **WINTER**
the season of nourishment, rest, preparation

Today's positive affirmation:
I am

Today I am grateful for:

Today's health and beauty goals:

**Beauty Nutrition
Essentials I Enjoyed Today:**

☐ Warm lemon water
☐ One or more servings of greens
☐ Seasonal fruit and veggies
☐ Protein and/or healthy fat
　at each meal
☐ Probiotics and/or fermented food
☐ Complete, mindful chewing at
　snack and mealtimes
☐ Fresh herbs and spices
☐ Regular meal intervals
☐ Frequent hydration
　(including ____ glasses of water)
☐ Supplements, if applicable
☐ Other:

**Self-Care Essentials
I Enjoyed Today:**

☐ Meditation and/or quiet time
☐ Deep breathing
☐ Physical activity
☐ Connection with friends
　or family
☐ De-stressing activity
☐ Self-love
☐ Beauty sleep (____ hours)
☐ Other:

DAILY FOOD DIARY

Breakfast
What I ate:

Time __:__ | Setting:

How I felt after eating:

Lunch
What I ate:

Time __:__ | Setting:

How I felt after eating:

Dinner
What I ate:

Time __:__ | Setting:

How I felt after eating:

Other
Today's snacks:

Favorite beauty foods I ate today:

_____ _____

_____ _____

_____ _____

_____ _____

When did you look and feel your best today?

_____

Takeaways from today:

DATE:

Current Season:

- ☐ **SPRING**
  the season of detox, renewal, lightening

- ☐ **SUMMER**
  the season of sun defense, hydration, activity

- ☐ **AUTUMN**
  the season of healing, balancing, grounding

- ☐ **WINTER**
  the season of nourishment, rest, preparation

Today's positive affirmation:
I am

Today I am grateful for:

Today's health and beauty goals:

Beauty Nutrition Essentials I Enjoyed Today:

- ☐ Warm lemon water
- ☐ One or more servings of greens
- ☐ Seasonal fruit and veggies
- ☐ Protein and/or healthy fat at each meal
- ☐ Probiotics and/or fermented food
- ☐ Complete, mindful chewing at snack and mealtimes
- ☐ Fresh herbs and spices
- ☐ Regular meal intervals
- ☐ Frequent hydration (including ____ glasses of water)
- ☐ Supplements, if applicable
- ☐ Other:

Self-Care Essentials I Enjoyed Today:

- ☐ Meditation and/or quiet time
- ☐ Deep breathing
- ☐ Physical activity
- ☐ Connection with friends or family
- ☐ De-stressing activity
- ☐ Self-love
- ☐ Beauty sleep (____ hours)
- ☐ Other:

DAILY FOOD DIARY

Breakfast
What I ate:

Time __:__   Setting:

How I felt after eating:

Lunch
What I ate:

Time __:__   Setting:

How I felt after eating:

Dinner
What I ate:

Time __:__   Setting:

How I felt after eating:

Other
Today's snacks:

Favorite beauty foods I ate today:

_____   _____

_____   _____

_____   _____

_____   _____

When did you look and feel your best today?

_____

Takeaways from today:

DATE:

Current Season:

☐ **SPRING**
the season of detox, renewal, lightening

☐ **SUMMER**
the season of sun defense, hydration, activity

☐ **AUTUMN**
the season of healing, balancing, grounding

☐ **WINTER**
the season of nourishment, rest, preparation

Today's positive affirmation:
I am

Today I am grateful for:

Today's health and beauty goals:

Beauty Nutrition Essentials I Enjoyed Today:

☐ Warm lemon water
☐ One or more servings of greens
☐ Seasonal fruit and veggies
☐ Protein and/or healthy fat at each meal
☐ Probiotics and/or fermented food
☐ Complete, mindful chewing at snack and mealtimes
☐ Fresh herbs and spices
☐ Regular meal intervals
☐ Frequent hydration (including ____ glasses of water)
☐ Supplements, if applicable
☐ Other:

Self-Care Essentials I Enjoyed Today:

☐ Meditation and/or quiet time
☐ Deep breathing
☐ Physical activity
☐ Connection with friends or family
☐ De-stressing activity
☐ Self-love
☐ Beauty sleep (____ hours)
☐ Other:

DAILY FOOD DIARY

Breakfast
What I ate:

Time __:__ | Setting:

How I felt after eating:

Lunch
What I ate:

Time __:__ | Setting:

How I felt after eating:

Dinner
What I ate:

Time __:__ | Setting:

How I felt after eating:

Other
Today's snacks:

Favorite beauty foods I ate today:

_____ _____

_____ _____

_____ _____

_____ _____

When did you look and feel your best today?

_____

Takeaways from today:

DATE:

Current Season:

- [ ] **SPRING**
  the season of detox, renewal, lightening
- [ ] **SUMMER**
  the season of sun defense, hydration, activity
- [ ] **AUTUMN**
  the season of healing, balancing, grounding
- [ ] **WINTER**
  the season of nourishment, rest, preparation

Today's positive affirmation:

I am

Today I am grateful for:

Today's health and beauty goals:

Beauty Nutrition Essentials I Enjoyed Today:

- [ ] Warm lemon water
- [ ] One or more servings of greens
- [ ] Seasonal fruit and veggies
- [ ] Protein and/or healthy fat at each meal
- [ ] Probiotics and/or fermented food
- [ ] Complete, mindful chewing at snack and mealtimes
- [ ] Fresh herbs and spices
- [ ] Regular meal intervals
- [ ] Frequent hydration (including ____ glasses of water)
- [ ] Supplements, if applicable
- [ ] Other:

Self-Care Essentials I Enjoyed Today:

- [ ] Meditation and/or quiet time
- [ ] Deep breathing
- [ ] Physical activity
- [ ] Connection with friends or family
- [ ] De-stressing activity
- [ ] Self-love
- [ ] Beauty sleep (____ hours)
- [ ] Other:

DAILY FOOD DIARY

Breakfast
What I ate:

Time __:__ | Setting:

How I felt after eating:

Lunch
What I ate:

Time __:__ | Setting:

How I felt after eating:

Dinner
What I ate:

Time __:__ | Setting:

How I felt after eating:

Other
Today's snacks:

Favorite beauty foods I ate today:

_____ _____

_____ _____

_____ _____

_____ _____

When did you look and feel your best today?

Takeaways from today:

DATE:

Current Season:

- [ ] **SPRING**
  the season of detox, renewal, lightening
- [ ] **SUMMER**
  the season of sun defense, hydration, activity
- [ ] **AUTUMN**
  the season of healing, balancing, grounding
- [ ] **WINTER**
  the season of nourishment, rest, preparation

Today's positive affirmation:

I am

Today I am grateful for:

Today's health and beauty goals:

Beauty Nutrition Essentials I Enjoyed Today:

- [ ] Warm lemon water
- [ ] One or more servings of greens
- [ ] Seasonal fruit and veggies
- [ ] Protein and/or healthy fat at each meal
- [ ] Probiotics and/or fermented food
- [ ] Complete, mindful chewing at snack and mealtimes
- [ ] Fresh herbs and spices
- [ ] Regular meal intervals
- [ ] Frequent hydration (including ＿＿ glasses of water)
- [ ] Supplements, if applicable
- [ ] Other:

Self-Care Essentials I Enjoyed Today:

- [ ] Meditation and/or quiet time
- [ ] Deep breathing
- [ ] Physical activity
- [ ] Connection with friends or family
- [ ] De-stressing activity
- [ ] Self-love
- [ ] Beauty sleep (＿＿ hours)
- [ ] Other:

DAILY FOOD DIARY

Breakfast
What I ate:

Time __:__ | Setting:

How I felt after eating:

Lunch
What I ate:

Time __:__ | Setting:

How I felt after eating:

Dinner
What I ate:

Time __:__ | Setting:

How I felt after eating:

Other
Today's snacks:

Favorite beauty foods I ate today:

_____ _____

_____ _____

_____ _____

_____ _____

When did you look and feel your best today?

_____

Takeaways from today:

DATE:

Current Season:

- [ ] **SPRING**
  the season of detox, renewal, lightening
- [ ] **SUMMER**
  the season of sun defense, hydration, activity
- [ ] **AUTUMN**
  the season of healing, balancing, grounding
- [ ] **WINTER**
  the season of nourishment, rest, preparation

Today's positive affirmation:
I am

Today I am grateful for:

Today's health and beauty goals:

Beauty Nutrition Essentials I Enjoyed Today:

- [ ] Warm lemon water
- [ ] One or more servings of greens
- [ ] Seasonal fruit and veggies
- [ ] Protein and/or healthy fat at each meal
- [ ] Probiotics and/or fermented food
- [ ] Complete, mindful chewing at snack and mealtimes
- [ ] Fresh herbs and spices
- [ ] Regular meal intervals
- [ ] Frequent hydration (including ____ glasses of water)
- [ ] Supplements, if applicable
- [ ] Other:

Self-Care Essentials I Enjoyed Today:

- [ ] Meditation and/or quiet time
- [ ] Deep breathing
- [ ] Physical activity
- [ ] Connection with friends or family
- [ ] De-stressing activity
- [ ] Self-love
- [ ] Beauty sleep (____ hours)
- [ ] Other:

DAILY FOOD DIARY

Breakfast
What I ate:

Time __:__ | Setting:

How I felt after eating:

Lunch
What I ate:

Time __:__ | Setting:

How I felt after eating:

Dinner
What I ate:

Time __:__ | Setting:

How I felt after eating:

Other
Today's snacks:

Favorite beauty foods I ate today:

_____ _____

_____ _____

_____ _____

_____ _____

When did you look and feel your best today?

_____

Takeaways from today:

DATE:

Current Season:

- [ ] **SPRING**
  the season of detox, renewal, lightening

- [ ] **SUMMER**
  the season of sun defense, hydration, activity

- [ ] **AUTUMN**
  the season of healing, balancing, grounding

- [ ] **WINTER**
  the season of nourishment, rest, preparation

Today's positive affirmation:
I am

Today I am grateful for:

Today's health and beauty goals:

Beauty Nutrition Essentials I Enjoyed Today:

- [ ] Warm lemon water
- [ ] One or more servings of greens
- [ ] Seasonal fruit and veggies
- [ ] Protein and/or healthy fat at each meal
- [ ] Probiotics and/or fermented food
- [ ] Complete, mindful chewing at snack and mealtimes
- [ ] Fresh herbs and spices
- [ ] Regular meal intervals
- [ ] Frequent hydration (including ____ glasses of water)
- [ ] Supplements, if applicable
- [ ] Other:

Self-Care Essentials I Enjoyed Today:

- [ ] Meditation and/or quiet time
- [ ] Deep breathing
- [ ] Physical activity
- [ ] Connection with friends or family
- [ ] De-stressing activity
- [ ] Self-love
- [ ] Beauty sleep (____ hours)
- [ ] Other:

DAILY FOOD DIARY

Breakfast
What I ate:

Time __:__ | Setting:

How I felt after eating:

Lunch
What I ate:

Time __:__ | Setting:

How I felt after eating:

Dinner
What I ate:

Time __:__ | Setting:

How I felt after eating:

Other
Today's snacks:

Favorite beauty foods I ate today:

_____ _____

_____ _____

_____ _____

_____ _____

When did you look and feel your best today?

_____

Takeaways from today:

A MOMENT TO CHECK IN

If you've reached this page, you've filled in ten journal entries. Take a moment to look back on what you've recorded and assess how your choices are impacting the way you look and feel. These questions will help you hone in on the foods and habits that are proving themselves to be most beneficial to your health and beauty, and point out adjustments that you may wish to make as you continue.

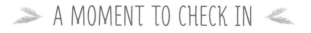

Describe the current state of your:

Skin	
Hair	
Nails	
Energy	
Weight	
Mood	
Resilience to Stress	

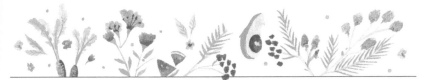

As you reflect on the previous journal entries, identify the following:

What new healthy habits did you cultivate during this period of journaling? What results did you see from these healthy habits?

Were there any new habits that didn't work well for you or didn't fit well into your lifestyle?

What challenges—including foods, thoughts, or habits—held you back from looking and feeling your best?

As you continue to build your new beautifying lifestyle, consider the following:

What are some new or developing beauty and health goals that you intend to focus on?

What are some challenges you foresee in the period ahead that might prevent you from meeting these goals?

Record words of encouragement or advice from yourself or others to inspire you along the way.

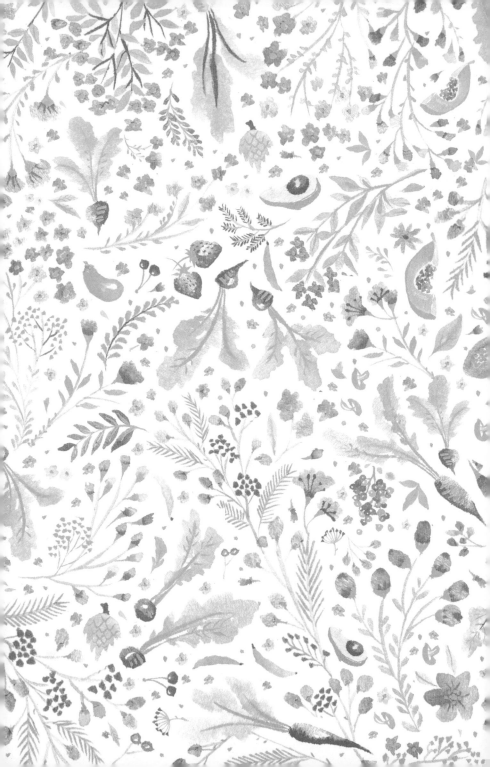

Conclusion

THE BEAUTY DOESN'T END HERE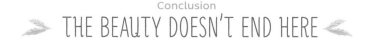

You've just set into motion a lifestyle that supports your healthiest, most beautiful self. From this moment on, I challenge you to build on this experience, apply what you've learned wherever life takes you, and return again and again to the specific practices that help you look and feel your absolute best. One of the more understated benefits of a lifestyle of beauty built around the seasons is that the calendar and the environment give you periodic reminders to check in with yourself and your needs. It's hard to stray too far before a seasonal shift gently reminds you to adjust your habits once more. Let each new season of the year and your life inspire you to reconnect with your beautifying routine. Going forward I hope you find—as you get dressed in the morning, cook a radiance-boosting dinner, or indulge in your favorite pampering activity—that you look and feel more beautiful, simply because you have the tools to be better cared-for, less stressed, and more deeply nourished—from the inside out.

ABOUT THE AUTHOR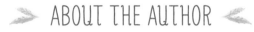

Jolene Hart, CHC, AADP, is a health coach certified by the Institute for Integrative Nutrition, a former magazine beauty editor, and founder of the pioneering beauty and health coaching practice Beauty Is Wellness (www.jolenehart.com). After resolving her own decade-long skin issues with changes to her diet and lifestyle, she began teaching women how to harness their power to transform their energy and appearance by making small, meaningful changes to their diet and self-care. Putting beauty nutrition to practice, she cooks, bakes, ferments, and blends from her kitchen in Philadelphia, PA, where she lives with her husband and son.